In the Labyrinth of Binge Eating

Hilda Dulin Lee

Journigan Publishing

All matters concerning your health require medical consultation with qualified health care professionals. This book is neither intended nor designed to replace the opinions of those professionals. Every effort has been made to give up-to-date information from credible sources; however, scientific information is constantly changing, so current information should always be consulted.

This book tells of Dr. Hilda Dulin Lee's personal journey through binge eating disorder. It is not intended to imply that others who binge eat will follow her pattern of behavior, nor necessarily solve their binge or weight problem using the techniques that worked for her.

First paperback edition, 2016
Journigan Publishing
Cedar Mountain, North Carolina

ISBN: 978-0-9969641-0-4
Library of Congress Control Number: 2015919945

To Glenn, the noblest person I know

and

To Patricia who taught me there is nobility in the struggle

ACKNOWLEDGMENTS

I want to thank Duke University's Diet and Fitness Center where I was first diagnosed with binge eating disorder, and especially Patricia Esperon, the counselor I saw there. As both counselor and friend, Patricia accompanied me on the journey I chronicle in this book and, without her, I'm not sure my healing, much less this book, would have been possible.

I also want to express appreciation to the University of North Carolina in Asheville where I was permitted to craft my Master's program around creative writing and research into binge eating. Dr. Melissa Himelein guided me in my research. Her unerring standards of good science, her breadth and depth of knowledge, and her openness and patience are all greatly appreciated.

I wish to thank all those I have met over the years who struggle along the same path I do and who have so generously shared their stories with me. We continue to learn from each other.

They say that friends help you move, but sisters help you move bodies. My sisters and I have moved some bodies—and even more ghosts—in the last several decades. There is no way I could have come to understand what I write of in this book without having shared my life's path with them and with my brother. My undying affection and appreciation go to all my siblings: Brenda, Dene, Jim, and Lynni.

I owe a debt of gratitude to the team of people who served as readers for this book as I shaped and proofed it. All of their suggestions and line editing made this a better book.

Finally, and most important of all, I want to acknowledge my husband, Glenn, who has stood by me through the best and the worst of times. He taught me how to love and to accept love. We celebrate our 50th anniversary this year and if we had another fifty years together, it would not be enough. He is the gentle love of my life who keeps me centered.

WHAT OTHERS HAVE SAID ABOUT THIS BOOK...

Hilda Lee has the mind of a scientist, the soul of an artist, and the voice of a gifted story-teller. She infuses the story of her own journey through binge eating with the latest research to produce a work of practical, useful art. This book is destined to touch the hearts and minds of thousands who binge eat as well as those who suffer from other addictions.— **Anonymous,** recovering binge eater

In the Labyrinth of Binge Eating is a major contribution to the literature on binge eating disorder. Many books have been written on the disorder, but only a small number with such power and honesty, by someone who has lived and struggled with the disorder. Hilda is fearless in sharing how her family history led to decades of soothing herself with food. She, like most people with the disorder, masked her deep feelings of shame and incompetence by pressing herself to be exceptional in all areas of her life. Readers will strongly identify with her unrelenting desire to be perfect, followed by her debilitating loss of control while bingeing. While Hilda's book serves as a powerful memoir about overcoming personal demons, it also describes effective strategies for dealing with binge eating. It is the gradual acceptance of herself as flawed and imperfect, yet still worthy of love, that is the most deeply healing aspect of her journey. Furthermore, the therapeutic strategies discussed are applicable to a number of mental health conditions such as PTSD, Anxiety, Depression, and Body Image. I cannot imagine a finer book to recommend to clients who are struggling with any of these issues. *In the Labyrinth of Binge Eating* is a powerful testament that with courage, compassion, and persistence, healing is possible.— **Patricia Esperon, Licensed Clinical Social Worker (LCSW)**

Hilda Lee presents a deeply honest account of the waxing and waning and eventual taming of binge-eating disorder (BED). Her vivid prose captures what it feels like to be in the body and mind of someone with BED. Some parts may evoke strong emotions, so readers should monitor their reactions and titrate exposure accordingly. Ultimately, Lee artfully illustrates her personal pathway to recovery and demonstrates that even when countless unexpected obstacles are thrown at one's feet, one can triumph over BED.— **Cynthia Bulik, PhD, FAED**, Founding Director of NC Center of Excellence for Eating Disorders & author of *Crave and Binge Control*.

Dr. Hilda Lee's book offers wonderful insights and suggestions about what it truly takes to recover from binge eating. It is captivating and offers a delicate balance between her own story and current research. I strongly recommend this book to my clients as well as treatment providers. Dr. Lee's practical and thoughtful suggestions and skill-building activities to break the cycle of binge eating are extremely helpful. Her T-I-C-K-E-T acronym is an amazing tool! This is a book about a healthy transformation that can help and inspire anyone who has felt stuck in a vicious cycle with food.—**Sofia Rydin-Gray, PhD, Licensed Psychologist**, Behavioral Health Director, Duke Diet and Fitness Center

There is nothing more compelling to someone who is struggling with an issue than a moving account from someone else who has suffered as they have and then conquered their demons. Hilda Lee begins *In the Labyrinth of Binge Eating* by taking us into the dark depths of her traumatic childhood and roots of her binge eating disorder. She chronicles in vivid detail what she did to soothe herself, the stifling shame she felt, the chronic dieting she did, the weight cycling her body endured, the desperate pursuit of over-achievement and perfection, and feelings of failure that plagued her throughout her life, until she finally sought the treatment that ended her struggle with BED. She catalogues the research she poured over to fully understand what was going on in her troubled brain and body and presents facts in a way that makes it all easy to understand. She shares the strategies she used to stop bingeing and heal herself. Best of all, Hilda's riveting narrative takes us with her on her journey to recovery, as if we're right there with her, cheering her on to an amazing transformation and affirmation of the strong, beautiful person she is, inside and out. Anyone who struggles with BED can find strength and hope in Hilda's story.— **Chevese Turner,** Founder, President, and CEO of Binge Eating Disorder Association (BEDA)

Contents

In the Labyrinth of Binge Eating

We have not even to risk the adventure alone; for the heroes of all time have gone before us; the labyrinth is thoroughly known; we have only to follow the thread of the hero-path. And where we had thought to find an abomination, we shall find a god; where we had thought to slay another, we shall slay ourselves; where we had thought to travel outward, we shall come to the center of our own existence.

Joseph Campbell
Hero with a Thousand Faces

How strange that all the terrors, pains, and early miseries,
Regrets, vexations, lassitudes interfused
Within my mind, should e're have borne a part,
And that a needful part, in making up
The calm existence that is mine when I
Am worthy of myself!

William Wordsworth
The Prelude: Book 1

In the Labyrinth of Binge Eating

~ x ~

Introduction

Shame

To others, I appeared to be a successful professional woman in complete control of my destiny. But I had a shameful secret. For most of my life, I was a compulsive, out-of-control binge eater. I secretly consumed massive amounts of food, at times unable to stop until I fell into a deep, almost coma-like sleep. At a top weight of more than 300 pounds, I suffered from high cholesterol, heart palpitations, back problems, chronic anxiety, and insomnia.

Far more devastating than this physical toll, however, was the crushing shame I felt for what I considered to be a major character flaw. Secretly, I was very much *out* of control, full of regret and shame, determined to keep this flaw hidden from everyone, especially from those I loved and respected.

Like most people who binge eat, I sought a solution to my problem in diet plans and weight loss books, thinking I simply needed to exert more will-power. Nothing could have been further from the truth. In fact, each diet I attempted not only took me further away from my weight-loss goal, but also led me deeper into the darkness of binge eating. I wandered in this maze of compulsive eating for more than forty years, struggling to find a way out, before I understood that bingeing was not really about food. Food was simply my drug of choice.

In 1998, as a last ditch effort to lose weight, I reluctantly went to a major weight-loss center for a month-long stay. There I was diagnosed with binge eating disorder (BED).

Binge eating disorder: recurring episodes of eating significantly more food in a short period of time than most people would eat under similar circumstances, with episodes marked by feelings of lack of control. The person may have feelings of guilt, embarrassment, or disgust and may binge eat alone to hide the behavior. This disorder is associated with marked distress and occurs, on average, at least once a week over three months.[1]

I did not realize it at the time, but many others share my plight. Binge eating disorder (BED) is more common than all other eating disorders combined (including anorexia and bulimia). More than 8 million Americans (5 million women and 3 million men) meet the clinical criteria for BED; many millions more do not meet the strict criteria but are, nonetheless, severely impacted by binge eating.[2]

In the Labyrinth of Binge Eating is the story of my journey back to physical and emotional health. Yes, I lost a great deal of weight over a period of several years, but my journey allowed me to release burdens far heavier than the fat I shed. Shame had crippled me and shame had kept me locked in a destructive, repetitive pattern of dieting, bingeing, and self-hatred. Letting go of shame was the greatest reward of my journey and was what allowed me to release many other destructive patterns in my life to embrace a joy that had previously been out of my reach. My recovery is so much more than the absence of bingeing.

But this book is more than my personal story; it also provides valuable information. My most fervent hope is that it informs and helps others who suffer as I did. Since 1994, when binge eating was first listed in the American Psychiatric Association's *Diagnostic and Statistical Manual of Mental Disorders (DMS-IV)* as a disorder in need of further study, and then in 2013 when it was designated as a distinct eating disorder in its own category,[3] much research has been done and much has been written in medical and social science journals concerning the disorder. Unfortunately, much of this powerful and helpful research remains buried in the scientific jargon of medical texts. It is still largely unavailable to those of us who binge. One of the goals of this book is to bring that valuable knowledge to the reader in a narrative form that is easily understood.

This book takes the reader from how it feels to be at the mercy of the binge beast to an understanding of what drives us into the labyrinth of binge eating in the first place to what to do in the moment of an intense craving, how to combat negative self-talk and how to find concrete solutions for everyday life. It also discusses personality patterns, like perfectionism and all-or-nothing thinking that keep us entrenched in this destructive pattern of eating. But this book covers more than just the struggle to overcome the behavior of binge eating; it also covers the incredible transformation that can occur because of that struggle.

I believe in the strength of the human spirit. Our struggles are often long and difficult; mine certainly has been. But there can be nobility in those struggles. I want to celebrate both the human spirit and the nobility we can find within ourselves as we struggle to heal and find our way back home again.

PART I

LOST IN THE LABYRINTH

There once lived a terrible beast: half man, half bull. This Minotaur lived in a deep dark cave on the Isle of Crete, isolated from the rest of the world by a complicated labyrinth.

Chapter One

Fractured View

1956 (age 9)

The heavy thud of Dad's bare feet on the linoleum floor awakens me. I sit up in bed. My heartbeat quickens and my chest tightens. I stare through the dark at the dim outline of the closed door that separates my bedroom from the kitchen—and from him. Suddenly the soft white light of the refrigerator illuminates the edges of the door. I creep out of bed, sit on the cold floor, and huddle in the darkness near the light. Through the crack at the hinge of the ill-fitting door, I watch my dad eat raw meat.

I pull my gown down around my legs and draw my knees in close to my chest. I don't want to watch, but I am pulled into his ritual. I sit mesmerized as he eats the bloody rump roast that was to be our family's Sunday dinner. After drinking hard liquor non-stop for several weeks and eating practically nothing, he now tears at the meat in silence, his face expressionless. The crack in the door allows me only a partial view, but I see more than I want to see. Blood drops from his mouth and hands and falls through his fingers, as if in slow motion, past his dingy sleeveless undershirt and filthy boxer shorts, past his pale bare legs, onto the top of his feet and to the floor where he stands. The dank stench of blood, body odor, and stale urine seeps through the crack in the door and hovers in the space between us.

From behind the door I continue to watch, my fractured

view revealing only broken slivers of this giant not four feet away. Waves of fear and revulsion wash over me. He eats chunks of the roast, leaving only bloody bits of mangled meat on the white butcher paper. He's finished now. His bloody hands smudge the white enamel crimson as he shuts the refrigerator door. The light goes out and we are both left in total darkness.

I listen to his muffled sobs as he makes his way across the room and slumps in his usual place at the head of the dinette table. Dad is an emotional man and I've heard him cry openly, but this sound is different. I'm ashamed to hear his private pain. I put my hands over my ears and imagine his usual cursing, but I cannot block out his weeping.

Once, when he whipped me for breaking a kaleidoscope, I tried not to make a sound. It wasn't my kaleidoscope, it was my sister's. How I loved to see its ever-changing, brightly-covered patterns.

"You never learn, do you, Hilda?" Dad said, as his leather belt stung my bare legs. I knew I would be punished, but fear of a whipping hadn't stopped me from taking the kaleidoscope apart. I had to see what was inside. It produced such glorious sights just by turning it round and round. What could be inside that caused such magnificent colors and patterns?

I cried long after the welts from Dad's whipping faded. I cried because all I found inside the kaleidoscope's wooden frame were ordinary bits and pieces of broken colored glass. I yearned for something more, something extraordinary, something exquisitely beautiful.

That was not the first, nor the last, whipping I suffered at the hands of my dad. Never an affectionate man, he was especially mean-spirited and violent when drunk. Where did his explosive anger come from? How can a man be filled with so much rage that he whips a child with a belt until welts rise? How can he give away his son's dog, then strike him when he cries? What drives a man to hit his wife because a phone rings too long? Then beat her almost unconscious when she cringes?

When we were young, the five of us kids never talked to each other about what went on in that house. Only when we were in our forties did we begin to understand that the anger and violence wasn't our fault: not Brenda's, my older sister, for her inability to control a chronic cough; not Dene's, my younger sister, for being such a nervous child; not Jim's, my younger brother, for failing to measure up to the memory of our half-brother Dan, killed in the Korean War before we could know him and before he could be a disappointment to Dad; not Lynni's, the baby of the family, for failing to keep the peace at all costs; and not mine for being imperfect, for not figuring out what I did that caused Dad's anger.

As children, we could no more stem the tide of violence and abuse inside that house than we could change the weather outside. But we kept on trying. And kept on feeling guilty for failing.

Dad's sobs die out. I take my hands from my ears and again pull my knees in close as I slowly rock back and forth. Shaky and slumped over, he smokes one Camel after another. By the glow of his cigarette, I see ashes drop to the floor. Years of fallen ashes have permanently grayed several of the white squares of the black-and-white linoleum. I hate those charred squares and have scrubbed and scrubbed them many times, but the stains won't go away, not even with steel wool and Ajax.

After stubbing out a last butt in his faded green oversized ashtray, Dad hunches over, putting his face in his hands. It doesn't matter that I can't see his face. The remembered image of his tortured features all but consumes me. In the middle of a drinking binge, Dad is always angry; he lashes out at whatever or whoever happens to be nearby. When he finally begins to sober up, though, that anger turns to sadness.

Sometimes it's a sloppy, wretched kind of sadness that only fills me with dread and disgust. But at other times, like tonight, it's a dark, heavy, anguished sorrow that's unbearable to witness. Finally, he stands up and slowly goes back toward his bedroom where Mom will pretend to be asleep.

Even though I know he'll fall asleep quickly after so much food (he always does), still I wait. Listening to my own fast, shallow breathing, I remain huddled by the door and wait. I look over at my younger sister in the bed we share. I can't see her in the dark, but the slow steady rhythm of her quiet breathing, and the soft whistle through her nose, tells me she's deep in sleep.

I can't leave the mess Dad has made. That would be evidence that things were not "normal" in our house. And so, as always, I sneak into the kitchen to begin one of the most dreaded tasks of my childhood. I must clean up after my dad so that no one, especially Mom, will have to see it in the morning. Mom may be weak and unable to help us, but we all know she's our only hope, so we protect her to protect ourselves.

I dare not turn on the light. I open the refrigerator, its dim bulb bright in the darkness, then turn to quietly lower the oven door. All of us kids fear Dad with a knife above all else, so when he's drinking, we hide knives away in various nooks and corners. I retrieve the sharp butcher knife from the back of the oven where I'd hidden it earlier.

I silently gag as I cut off the gnawed parts of the meat and quietly rewrap what's left of the roast. With a soiled dishrag, already stiff from filth, I wipe the blood from the refrigerator and the floor. I hide the dirty rag and the bloody knife under the sink behind the garbage pail. I don't turn on the water faucet; the knocking of the old pipes might wake the others. I'll wash the rag and knife tomorrow.

I quietly lift Dad's chair and place it back under the edge of the table, clean up his ashes and butts, and straighten the top of the counter. I look around the kitchen. All is back to normal. I can return to bed.

But as I start to push the refrigerator door shut, I spot the banana pudding that Mom made for Sunday dessert. A strong urge to eat comes over me. I want something cool and soft. I can carefully lift the meringue, scoop up one spoonful from under the edge, and then replace the meringue layer. No one will ever notice. I'm good at that sort of thing. One bite won't matter. I take the pudding out of the fridge and sit by the table on the grayed linoleum. That first spoonful brings comfort to an ache I cannot name. The pudding is so smooth, so cool, so soft. I take another spoonful. And another. And another. With each bite, the ache I cannot name recedes just a little, and my craving for more grows stronger and stronger. I keep going, urged on by an ancient instinct that takes me to a deep, dark, comforting place. Before I know it, the entire pudding is gone. And so is the elusive sadness that I felt. In fact, I taste and feel nothing now. Nothing but a blessed emptiness—and an uncontrollable desire for more. My quiet eating frenzy continues with a half jar of Peter Pan peanut butter and what's left of a loaf of Merita bread. I leave the Saltine crackers on the counter. Too loud.

Numb and tired, I hide the empty containers at the bottom of the garbage can, the pudding bowl and spoon under the sink with the knife and rag, and I creep back into bed. I fall into a deep coma-like sleep. No one—not Mom, not any of my three sisters, not my brother—will know what I've done. They'll silently blame Dad for the missing food. There are so many secrets in this house, under beds and in dark corners. What is one more?

The next morning I'm ashamed. Ashamed of stealing food from my family. Ashamed of being a glutton. Ashamed of being the fattest kid in my grade. But most unbearable is the shame of being the shadow of my dad, sneaking around and eating like an animal.

Please, God, forgive me just this one more time. Make me strong and pure. I promise I'll never steal food again. I'll never eat sweets again as long as I live. I'll be good. I'll be strong. I'll be perfect.

And I *was* perfect—for almost a month. In that month I ate practically nothing. I washed the dishes and cleaned the floors and polished the furniture. I studied even harder than usual, and would accept nothing less than an A+. But perfection is a hard task master. Something inevitably goes wrong. Giving in to a cookie or missing a question on an arithmetic test meant total failure. I was either perfect or I was worthless. These cycles of perfection and failure, of starving and bingeing, continued for decades before I could see more than the fractured view from behind the door.

1998 (age 51)

I shook my head in disbelief as I looked closely at the building where I would spend all of my waking hours for the next month. My difficult decision to come to this place had been well-researched and well-thought out, but now I was beginning to question the wisdom of my decision. The bright blue awnings over the doors and windows couldn't camouflage the dreariness of the old brick building. How could this mundane, outmoded building, in a poor, unkempt section of town, house Duke University's Diet and Fitness Center? This was supposed to be one of the best medically supervised weight reduction programs in the country. A place where the really desperate and medically compromised came for help. It was nothing like I had imagined. Where were the tree-lined shady streets? The beautiful stone gothic buildings? The bustling team of white-coated experts who would guide me to the promised land of health and beauty? The building I approached looked more like a junior high school from the 1960s. For what I was paying to be probed and prodded, fed and exercised, things should have looked a lot more appealing, more modern, more promising.

I did not easily ask for help. I was a self-made and independent woman. I took great pride in being able to troubleshoot any problem and come up with the perfect solution. And yet here I stood, admitting defeat over my own body. I didn't want to be here, but more than a year earlier, I'd made a pact with myself. If, after one year (I marked the date in my new Franklin planner), I was unable to lose, and keep off, at least 60 pounds, I would seek professional help. I would go to a major residential weight-loss center like this one.

But guess what? The year had come and gone, and I weighed more than ever. I'd dragged myself through each day, pretending to be the strong and efficient wife, mother, sister, daughter, and dentist that I was supposed to be. Pact or no pact, it wasn't a good time to keep the "selfish" promise I'd made earlier. My mother was slowly dying and required around-the-clock care, which my siblings and I provided on top of our full-time jobs. We were blessed to be able to keep her at home, but it was a grueling time for all of us. At work, one of the dentists in my practice left with little notice. This put an additional load on the rest of us. I was dipping into the last of my reserves of time, energy, and sheer will. Exhausted and depressed, I was at the end of my rope. Then something happened that pushed me well beyond my ability to rebound.

My adult son and his three-year-old twin boys were in an automobile accident that left one of the twins in a coma. For five days, Michael clung to life, and for five days, family members clung to one another. On the fifth day, Michael woke up, and by the seventh was back home. Within a few weeks, he was the bright, active, inquisitive child he'd been before the accident. To see him now, you'd never know how close to death he'd come.

That week, however, broke me. I'd dozed only a few minutes during those five days and nights. When the crisis was over, I slept for eighteen hours, but woke up still exhausted. I struggled to function at all. Thoughts seemed scattered and wouldn't congeal; the smallest action required unavailable strength. Fighting to hold my emotions in check, I was overwhelmed with a sense of vulnerability, a sense that no one I knew and loved would ever be safe again. I'd survived breast cancer several years earlier but, even then, I hadn't felt as helpless or hopeless as this.

Stoically, I forced myself back to work within days after Michael left the hospital. I tried to push my anxiety and physical exhaustion into a corner. I did nothing but work and eat. Lots and lots of eating. My sleep was sporadic at best. I developed an erratic heartbeat. I knew that stress and excess weight put me at risk for a heart attack, but mostly I feared a recurrence of the cancer. I was fully aware that stress and trauma could lower the immune system and allow any lurking cancer cells to grow and reproduce. That fear is what drove me to my oncologist for testing.

There were no signs of a recurrence, but he shared my concern. "You better find a way to relax, or your body will find it for you," he said. Then he sent me to my internist for a complete physical.

After labs and an exam, my internist said what almost every doctor I'd ever seen had said, "What you need is to lose some weight. You simply cannot keep going in the direction you're going and expect to see your grandkids grow up. You won't make it to sixty if you don't change your ways. You're a bright woman. Why can't you see that your lifestyle is going to kill you? And soon."

And so, with great trepidation, I left my dental practice in the hands of others, and my share of caring for Mom to my already over-loaded siblings. I made my way to North Carolina where the weight-loss center I had chosen was located. I hated admitting I needed help. And I hated burdening others with duties that were rightfully mine. Shirking responsibility simply wasn't in my nature. Everything in me rebelled at the decision I was forced to make. And yet I didn't know what else to do.

As I stared at the building in front of me, I tried to focus on hope. The faint, desperate hope that this place would provide the help I needed. But the best I could muster was embarrassment and a pervasive sadness that I had come to this. I wished it had been rainy and cold to match my spirit that day in February, but the sun shone in defiance of my mood.

I trudged up the steps of the building, nervously clutching the bulging folder that housed my massive medical history, a history that had grown exponentially over the last decade. I also carried an intrusive fifteen page questionnaire that I'd loathed filling out. The questions seemed irrelevant and humiliating. I'd cringed as I responded to questions such as:

- Do you hide food and eat it later in secret?
- Do you spill food on yourself when you eat?
- Were you ever physically or sexually abused?
- Do you ever have thoughts or fantasies of suicide?
- Are you comfortable with your body?
- Do you like your body?

Oh, sure, I like this mass of flesh I drag around every day! Besides, what has any of this got to do with my weight??

I had lied about my maximum weight on the form. I couldn't bear for anyone to know I'd hit 298 pounds before I stopped weighing altogether. I had no idea what my max weight was, but I knew it was well over 300 pounds. I'd answered the rest of the behavioral questionnaire honestly, but was set to leave if they started in with any psychological mumbo-jumbo. I was here for one purpose and one purpose only: to get a head start on losing a lot of weight so I could get on with my busy, productive life.

At least I was proud of one form in the folder, and that was the food diary. It documented all that I'd eaten for the last ten days, which wasn't much. It was accurate, but hardly a fair accounting of my usual food intake. I'd starved myself for much of January in a last ditch effort to shed some weight. *Please don't let me be the fattest person there.* I didn't think I could bear to be the fattest person at a "fat farm." I was far from it, as I would soon discover.

I took a deep breath, mustered my resolve, and walked into the building. After orientation and a short introductory tour, the ten of us who were new arrivals joined about fifty or so regular participants in the cafeteria line in the dining hall. I was delighted—and guilty to be delighted—to see I was *not* the fattest. In fact, I clearly weighed less than most people in the room. Even though there was a range of sizes and shapes, a significant number were extremely heavy; some so heavy that they could only walk with the aid of walkers.

I was in line behind a rather pretty twenty-something year-old blonde who must have weighed close to 400 pounds. She not only used a walker, but also dragged an oxygen tank along beside her. Her heavy breathing told me how difficult it was for her just to get her meal. She looked at my name tag, smiled the kindest smile I'd ever seen, and said in a heavy Texas drawl, "You're new, aren't you? The first week is tough, finding your way around and all. But it gets easier."

"How long have you been here?"

"Almost seven weeks."

Seven weeks! That seemed like an awful long time to learn the simple skills of eating and exercise. I even thought the four weeks I'd committed to stay was unreasonably long. I wanted to talk to her more, but we both had our trays of food. She sat down in the main dining hall, but I had to report to a back room where the new incoming group was to meet.

I later learned that many of the participants had diabetes, heart disease, and other chronic illnesses. I wavered between gratitude for my own reasonably good health and horror at seeing myself in a few years if this program didn't work for me. It felt both comfortable and embarrassing to be in the presence of so many others who were severely obese.

The first few days were a blur. Between a complete medical exam, appointments with a nutritionist, an exercise expert, and a psychologist, and classes on food, meal planning, and exercise, my head was spinning. The staff's level of knowledge impressed me, and I was pleased that we were treated as intelligent, successful people. I thought everything was going pretty well until the fourth day when I received a note that made me blanch.

It basically said that the answers to the entrance questionnaire I'd filled out indicated that I had a binge eating problem, and that I should attend the series of classes on binge eating the following Monday, Wednesday, and Friday. I knew what the note meant—that I was being forced into a remedial class because I was such a slob. I wished I'd been a little less truthful on the questionnaire. I knew I ate a lot of food, but I certainly wasn't a "binge" eater. The word *binge* had a terrible association for me. It took me back to my dad's binge drinking, and I wanted no connection to that world. I decided I would attend the class just once, but I had no intention of wasting my time three times a week on a class I didn't need.

It turned cool and the rain poured the following Monday. Even the gods knew better than to let the sun shine that day! I sneaked into the back dining room where the binge class was to be held. As the first person there, I had my choice of seats. I sat near the back row, in a corner, determined to prove them wrong. *I do not belong in this class. I am not like my dad.*

In filed about twenty other people, some men, but mostly women. Some were quiet and looked embarrassed, but others chatted as if this were just another class. Finally, the instructor walked in and shut the door. I quickly sized her up. A beautiful short-haired brunette, she was impeccably dressed in a beige linen knee-length straight skirt and a pale green blouse, neatly tucked in around her small waist. Her easy smile and confident manner communicated a sense of kind authority. She appeared athletic, as if she could run a marathon with ease. She also looked quite young, but I saw from her name tag that she had a Ph.D.

After everyone took a seat, she introduced herself as Anne. She explained this would be an interactive class. "It only works if we're all honest and open."

I, for one, would not be "open." I would not, in fact, be participating at all. I did not need to be in this class. My time would be far better spent in the gym or in a class on some medical issue.

"So, let's get started," Anne said. "This is a class on binge eating. What do you think binge eating is?" she asked the class as she walked to the shiny whiteboard and picked up a green marker. Finally, an annoyed-looking man in his forties spoke.

"I don't know why I'm in this class," he said. "I thought binge eating was where you ate a lot of food and then vomited, but I've never vomited after eating, unless I was sick."

"You're actually half right," said Anne. "Binge eating *is* eating a lot of food, but it's a myth that most binge eating is followed by some form of purging, such as vomiting or the use of laxatives. Bingeing *and* purging is found in an eating disorder called bulimia nervosa, which carries its own special medical risks. There are far more people, however, who binge and *don't* purge than those who do. Many of you binge, and to an extent that it severely affects your lives, but few, if any, of you purge. If you do purge and have not already addressed this with the staff, please come and talk with me or one of the other counselors."

Anne paused a moment. "Any other questions about the purging issue?"

When no one responded, Anne wrote **LARGE AMOUNT OF FOOD** on the whiteboard.

"So bingeing is eating a lot of food. What do you call a lot of food?" Anne asked.

Slowly and reluctantly, the people in the class began to list their binge food and the quantities. I kept quiet.

"A large bag of chips."

"A gallon of ice cream."

"A bag of chips *and* a gallon of ice cream!"

The class laughed. Tension eased.

"A large sausage and pepperoni pizza. Extra cheese."

"A pan of lasagna."

"A whole chocolate pie."

More people joined in as the class became emboldened, and seemingly relieved, to finally speak the unspeakable. I was embarrassed for them. And for myself. I had, on many occasions, eaten most of what they called out.

"A dozen doughnuts."

"A box of Little Debbie cakes."

"Hell, I've eaten four Whoppers and three large fries at once," said a giant bearded man.

There was a break in the comments when a shy-looking woman in front of me spoke. "My three-year-old son's birthday cake," she said somberly. I saw red creep up the folds in the back of her neck. "Can you imagine? I ate my son's birthday cake, and the bakery was closed, so there was no cake for his party."

I remembered my family's banana pudding. I felt sick. Shamed.

"I once ate a chicken casserole I made for a dying neighbor," a huge elderly black woman with thin white hair said.

The room grew quieter. We had moved into new territory now.

"We had a barbeque planned at my house once," an extremely overweight woman with a strong New Jersey accent said. "I ate two dozen brownies as soon as I made them. I called my husband at work and told him to stop by the bakery. I lied and said I'd burnt the brownies."

My cheeks burned. I had lied about food I'd eaten many times.

A tall massive red-headed woman, who had been quiet until now, spoke up. "I don't discriminate," she said softly. "I'll eat absolutely anything when I'm in that state."

Anne turned to the woman. "Describe that 'state' you're talking about."

The woman hesitated, nervously fingering her brightly-painted nails. "When I binge, it feels like...like I'm not in control anymore. Once I start, I can't stop."

"Yeah!" Several people spoke at once, and others nodded.

"Like I'm possessed!"

I thought my heart would burst right out of my chest. *Oh my God! That's me. Possessed! That's what it feels like.*

The heaviest woman in the room spoke my thoughts. "All I can think of is to get to food. Sometimes a particular food; sometimes anything will do."

Anne nodded and smiled. "Ok, class, you have just defined binge eating."

She gracefully moved across the shiny tiled floor to a stand that held a flip chart and opened it to a page that gave a definition.

Binge eating: eating an inappropriately large quantity of food in a relatively short period of time, accompanied by a feeling of having lost control.

A short nervous man with the thickest neck I'd ever seen raised his hand. "I stuff myself every year at Thanksgiving." His voice was rough and gravelly. "It tastes so good I don't *want* to stop, but I feel like I *could* stop if I wanted to. Are you saying that's not a binge?"

"That's correct, it's not a binge. At least not by the strict clinical definition." Anne went on to explain that most people overeat at one time or another, especially at holidays, but it's not a binge if the person doesn't experience an overwhelming feeling that they can't stop.

"Conversely," Anne said, "some people may lose control, and eat more than they feel they should, but not enough to be considered an inappropriate amount by normal standards. A good example of this would be what a person with anorexia might experience. That type of out-of-control eating," she explained, "is not a true binge because it doesn't meet both criteria."

Anne described just how much food was sometimes consumed in a single binge. She said that some people may eat as much as *twenty* or even *thirty* times the recommended daily allowance of calories, although that amount was unusually large for a binge. I did some quick figuring in my head. That had to be over 30,000 calories! I calculated that I'd eaten as many as 10,000 or 15,000 calories at a time, but 30,000??

Anne broke my train of thought. "The big difference between simply stuffing oneself and bingeing is not just in the actual amount of food consumed, but rather in the state of mind that accompanies the overeating." She moved back to the whiteboard and below the words **LARGE AMOUNT OF FOOD**, she wrote **LOSS OF CONTROL**.

"This significant element of having lost control is central to understanding binge eating." She circled the words she had just written. "In fact, the binge often continues until the food is all gone, or until the binger is so uncomfortable that he or she cannot consume anything else and falls asleep from exhaustion."

I shifted uncomfortably in my seat. I knew that kind of sleep. I'd gone there often.

"Ok, so now we know what binge eating is. Let's continue by talking more about how it *feels* when you binge."

Silence. Finally the red-head spoke. "What do you mean, how it feels?"

"Well, let's start at the beginning. What does it feel like when you take that first bite at the beginning of what turns out to be a binge?"

Anne nodded for the red-head to continue.

"I don't know. I guess maybe a sense of relief more than anything. Relief to finally just give in to the incredibly strong urge."

"It's more than relief for me," the pretty blonde I'd met the first day drawled. I hadn't even noticed she was in the class until she spoke. "I feel a sense of euphoria. My brother is an alcoholic, and I think it may be similar to what he describes when he finally gives in to that first drink after a long period of sobriety. Just sweet euphoria."

A short, round woman in a bright orange sweat suit spoke next. "The first bite is wonderful. I feel soothed and comforted. Anxiety just disappears. Everything is kind of quiet and calm and slowed down. Nothing matters but the feeling the food gives me."

"Yeah, I know exactly what you're talking about. I slowly savor that first bite or two," a woman in the front row added. "But then I start eating faster and faster."

"Oh, for sure!" Phyllis, one of the people who had come in Sunday with my group, said. "I get into a sort of eating frenzy, where the food just flies into my mouth. It seems like my eating accelerates as the binge goes on."

Anne wrote key words on the board as people spoke.

"What else?" she prompted.

"After a while, I don't feel anything, don't even taste the food anymore. I just feel numb."

"Disconnected. Unplugged."

Comments were coming from all around the room.

"Yes! That's it!" a young blonde said. "I don't feel good or bad. It's not that it's pleasant. In fact, I don't feel any pleasure at all at that point."

"And no pain either," someone chimed in. "I think that void, that disconnection is what I'm after all along. That numbing that bingeing brings."

Anne spoke. "This numb feeling you're talking about is quite common. As the binge continues, almost everyone says they begin to feel numb, no longer tasting the food, and feeling emotionally anesthetized as well." She explained that those who binge learn through experience that this anesthetic quality blocks negative emotions of all kinds and, as such, becomes a major motivator for the continuance of this eating behavior. She ended her explanation with "Some people even report an altered state of consciousness, a feeling of dissociation."

Dissociation. I would never have thought to use that word in relation to bingeing, but it was perfect. I thought of the use of the word in my chemistry classes in college. I vaguely remembered the definition as a process whereby a molecule is split into simpler groups of atoms. *That's the feeling. That's what I yearn for as I get lost in the food. I want to split apart from myself.*

I wanted to explore that idea further, but Anne's voice interrupted my thoughts and brought my attention back to the classroom. I didn't want to miss a thing.

"Let's talk a minute about *how* you binge. Alone? With others? In front of the television? That sort of thing."

Much of the bashfulness in the group was gone now. Several people spoke up at the same time.

"Oh, always alone. I would never let anyone see me eat like that."

"Definitely alone. Always in secret."

"Yes, alone. And either standing at the kitchen counter or in front of the television."

"I can really zone out all by myself with food and TV."

"Occasionally," Anne said, "I'll meet a person who has a

'binge partner,' but most people binge alone and in secret. Why do you think that is?"

"I would be so ashamed if anyone knew," said the shy lady who had eaten her son's birthday cake.

"Yes," Anne said. "Binge eating is almost always associated with a great deal of guilt and shame."

Oh, the shame! All the shame, for all the years, came flooding in. Tears rolled down my cheeks. Through my sobs, I spoke up for the first time. "I sometimes feel worthless for being so weak. For failing yet again. Guilty and ashamed of hiding food and sneaking around. Terrified I'll be found out."

Anne's eyes teared up slightly as she walked to the side of the room where I sat. "That feeling of shame takes a huge toll on self-esteem," she said. "It may be the most destructive aspect of binge eating. And it is something we'll talk a lot about in the up-coming meetings."

Anne directed our attention to the board where she'd been writing as we talked. "Look at these words. They pretty much cover the major elements of binge eating."

LARGE AMOUNT OF FOOD
LOSS OF CONTROL
RELIEF
EUPHORIA
SOOTHED & COMFORTED
FRENZIED & ACCELERATED
ALONE
IN SECRET
NUMB
DISCONNECTED
SHAME & GUILT

"I want to clarify a point that's sometimes confusing for our clients," Anne said. She then explained that if a person binges, on average, at least once a week over a three month period and doesn't use any form of purging, he or she is classified as having *binge eating disorder*.[1]

"About 3% to 5% of all adults in the U.S., and up to 40% of participants at treatment centers such as ours here, meet the requirements for that diagnosis," Anne said. "We, however, along with many other researchers and clinicians, feel that it's a somewhat arbitrary classification. We see a huge range of bingeing patterns. Some clients report bingeing that occurs in distinct episodes that last for one sitting, and may not be repeated for long periods of time. Others have binge episodes that last for months, with massive eating occurring every day."

That's me, I thought. My binge episodes would continue for months on end, with each day filled with eating as much as my body could possibly hold, ending with a weight gain of forty, fifty, even sixty or seventy pounds.

Anne continued. "Binge eating falls on a continuum as far as weight and bingeing behavior is concerned. Some normal weight and mildly overweight people report difficulties with binge eating, but the level of obesity goes up dramatically as the frequency and the severity of bingeing increases. Also, people don't usually start off with full-blown binge eating disorder, but may progress gradually from mild weight preoccupation to occasional bouts of compulsive over-eating to a more serious form in which daily life is completely disrupted. Many people fall in and out of the classification as they swing between bingeing and periods of normal eating. Whether you meet the specific criteria for binge eating disorder isn't really the issue. How often or how long you binge is not nearly as important as how you're *affected* by it. If bingeing is negatively affecting your life and your health, we're concerned. And we're here to help."

Anne paused to allow for any questions, but there were none. "I hope to see all of you again on Wednesday," she said as she dismissed the class.

Before this class, I truly had denied that I had anything more than a weakness for food. I knew I overate. I knew I preferred eating alone, and that I often hid how much I ate from others. I knew that food gave me great comfort. And afterward I felt great shame. But I hadn't really seen the pattern before. Just bits and pieces. And I certainly hadn't known there were a great many other people like me. And yet here they were, people who shared the same secret.

My classmates struggled to their feet and shuffled out of the room. These people knew what it felt like to be possessed, to be driven to eat to exhaustion. They knew about getting lost in food in order to feel numb. Most important of all, they had felt the same horrible shame that I'd felt. And we had actually talked about it. I'd come here for help with my obesity, but clearly I was not going to be able to deal with that obesity without also dealing with the behavior of binge eating.

Binge eating disorder. It felt good to be able to name it. And to admit to it. Maybe now I could learn to understand it. And eventually beat it.[2]

On Wednesday, I went into class and sat in the front row. I resolved to learn whatever I had to learn, and to change whatever I had to change, in order to destroy this monster that was trying to destroy me. I would take my sword and slay the beast! Little did I know the path my journey would take. Or that, in the end, my sword would be of little value.

PART II

RETRACING THE PATH

To keep the terrible Minotaur appeased and safely hidden away in the cave, young boys and girls were regularly sent to be sacrificed. It was a heart-breaking ritual for the people of Athens. Many families lost their beautiful young children, and the community lost its best and brightest.

While hundreds of strong warriors died in their efforts to find and slay the creature, hope was restored when Theseus decided to challenge the depths of the cave and confront the Minotaur. He diligently prepared for his dangerous journey into the labyrinth, not knowing what he would find in its depths.

"I will destroy the beast!" boldly shouted young Theseus as he polished his armor and sharpened his sword.

Chapter Two

Shadows on the Wall: The Unsafe Child

"What do you remember about that Christmas in Sparkman Homes?" my sister, Brenda, asked. I picked a small nut out of my cranberry-walnut muffin and chewed it longer than necessary. I sipped the last of my tea, then sighed deeply. *So, we're all finally going to talk about it after more than forty years.*

Since 1999, my three sisters and I had met once a year for our "sisters' week-end." Brenda, Dene, Lynni and I had been laughing and playing games the whole week-end. Our time together came but once a year and we always made the most of it, catching up on each other's lives and competing at Monopoly as ferociously as we did when we were children.

Now a quiet heaviness settled over the room. We all knew which Christmas Brenda meant. Through the years, some of us, one-on-one, had broached the edges of the subject, but never before had all four sisters put it out on the table. For the next five hours, there in Brenda's kitchen, we shared the most indelibly etched memory of our childhood.

1958

I gripped the neck of the green coca-cola bottle hidden beneath the folds of my ragged skirt. Not much protection, but all I had. The five of us Dulin kids sat like statues on the worn brown sofa and stared at the butcher knife Dad held near Mom's throat.

Outside, darkness settled over the alleys of Sparkman Homes, the low-rent housing project where we lived. Inside, the only lamp in the room cast Dad's giant shadow on the dingy concrete block wall across from him.

Don't move. Don't blink. Don't breathe.

Our safety that night was fragile, and could be blown away with the least puff of air.

Mom sat across from us in the straight-back chair that Dad had dragged into the middle of the room, her stubby hands neatly folded in her lap. Her apron, so faded you couldn't tell what color it had once been, covered the front of her blue print dress. At her feet was a dishrag she'd dropped when Dad grabbed her. Scattered beside it were the Lennon Sisters paper dolls my two younger sisters had been playing with.

Mom remained passive and offered no resistance as Dad's huge hand grabbed her by the hair and pulled her head back. He pressed the knife against her neck. The knife with the dark brown handle and the large sharp blade. The one I'd failed to hide. *It's all my fault.*

As always, when Dad's violence mounted, we followed the rules. Be very still and make no sound. Don't even breathe. Show no emotion. Disappear into yourself so he can't see you. But stay vigilant, ready.

"Look what your mother has brought me to!" Hatred roughened his voice, words were slurred from whiskey, but the message was clear. "I'm gonna cut off her God-damned head and y'all can watch it roll across the floor."

For the first few hours, all he'd done was yell and curse, but it had escalated to the butcher knife. Sometimes, when the worst violence came, my older sister, Brenda, could take the youngest ones to hide in the pantry or a closet while I stayed with Mom to face Dad. Tonight, though, Dad kept us all together, ordering us to sit on the sofa.

I tightened my grip on the coca-cola bottle and prayed he would pass out. I waited in controlled terror, perfectly still, my breathing shallow and even, trying not to disturb even one molecule of air. *Should I intercede? Or should I wait and hope he passes out before he kills Mom and then us?* The weight of that decision pressed in on me.

Suddenly Dad staggered away from Mom and over to the skimpy Christmas tree in the corner. The icicles swung from the dry pine like tiny slivers of metal; the red balls bobbed as Dad's shoulder brushed against the branches; dried pine needles dropped to the floor beneath. He leaned his forehead against the wall, taking labored breaths. For a moment, I thought he might pass out and drop the knife.

But he didn't. Instead, he stumbled back toward us, knocking over the table lamp. The bent shade tumbled and bumped awkwardly across the floor while the rest of the lamp dangled upside down by its cord. The bare bulb, still intact, still shining, glared accusingly at me. Had I missed my chance to act? Again he put the knife to Mom's jugular. I had not fully understood that word when we learned it in science class, but now, as I saw the blood pulsing in my mother's *jugular*, I got it.

"You sorry God-damned bitch! Why you makin' me do this?"

Spit drooled from the corners of Dad's mouth. He was tiring, his jaws softening, going slack. He lowered the knife and staggered across the room to the dinette table several feet away. Slumping down in his chair, he placed the knife onto the formica table. He fumbled with a cigarette pack until he shook one out. He lit it, took several long draws, and stared at us through rheumy eyes. We all remained frozen. No air stirred in the room. *Pass out. Pass out.*

Dad's eyelids drooped and his head bobbed and jerked, trying to stay conscious. *Pass out. Please pass out.* Eventually, he slumped over, lit cigarette falling to the floor. The danger was passing. In a few minutes, he slowly wobbled to his feet, eyes half-open, and stumbled to his bedroom where he would sleep for many hours.

Rising stiffly from her chair without saying a word or changing her distant expression, Mom moved slowly and mechanically. Our cue. All five of us stood up. In unison. As if a choir director had lifted his hands for all to rise.

We went silently about our unspoken and unassigned, yet very clear, tasks. We each knew our role. As if we had thoroughly read and rehearsed a school play. Mom stepped on the cigarette to put it out, then went into the bedroom and pulled the covers up over Dad; Brenda put Lynni and Jim to bed on the sofa; Dene and I straightened up, putting the chair and the lamp and its shade back in place.

With everything in order, the room looked normal once again. As if nothing at all had happened. Except for the butcher knife which still lay on the dinette table. I carefully retrieved the knife and placed it in the sink, hiding it under dirty pots soaking in cold, greasy water.

Brenda and Mom joined me in the kitchen. Mom's hollow voice feigned cheerfulness as it broke through the deafening quiet. "Let's finish making these desserts."

Staring out at the darkness, in a flat, emotionless monotone, she told us, "This will be the best Christmas ever. A special Christmas."

And so we prepared for the Christmas season. While Mom mashed sweet potatoes for a pie, Brenda and I iced the carrot cake. Working on opposite sides of the cake, we were careful not to let our spatulas touch, or our eyes meet.

Brenda remembered what Mom told her that night: "Don't worry. In a few years none of you will remember any of this."

Not remember? Here we sat, more than forty years later, able to retrace almost every movement, to recall almost every sentence. And during all these intervening years, not one of us has kept any large sharp knives in our homes. That Christmas in Sparkman Homes was indeed *special*.

1998

My heart pounded; my breath came quick and shallow between sobs; my hands sweaty, my mouth dry. I slumped in a chair, hiding in a back hall where I hoped I wouldn't be seen. I sobbed uncontrollably as each new wave of anxiety engulfed me. It was the third week of my stay at Duke's Diet and Fitness Center.

A single piece of paper, a paper I'd lost three hours earlier, a simple form I was to turn in that morning—that's what had set off this inescapable, uncontrollable onslaught of emotion. It wasn't a big deal. A new form was easily obtainable from the office. But it *felt* like a big deal.

You stupid idiot! An inner voice screamed. *You can't do anything right. You can't even muster enough will power to lose weight on your own. That's why you had to practically commit yourself to this place. And now you can't even keep track of a simple piece of paper? How do you even function in the world?*

I'd managed to get myself dressed and to the first class, but I couldn't stop the chatter in my head. When no one sat next to me, I knew why. *No one really likes you. Face it. Do you have any real friends? Sure, you have patients who pay you; you have employees paid to tolerate you; you have family obligated to care about you. But here, you can see yourself as the loser you are. You're nothing. You're nobody. No one even wants to be near you.*

I left the class before it started and found an out-of-the-way hall in which to hide.

The feelings of dread and self-loathing just wouldn't stop. Wave after wave. I thought I would have a heart attack. Between peaks of anguish, I kept asking myself why I felt so out-of-control. After all, I was normally a got-it-together sort of woman, a pillar of strength that others could always depend on. I rarely lost control of my emotions. Even with that wicked voice in my head condemning me at every turn, I always held it together and pushed forward. So why not here? Why not now?

The answer finally came, and with it a new devastation. No, this wouldn't have happened back home. Long before reaching this level of intense anxiety, I'd have soothed the savage beast with food. I'd realized for a long time that I ate my way through major stress, but until that moment, sitting alone and sobbing in the hall, I had no idea of the extent to which I used food for comfort.

Back home, I wouldn't have fretted over a lost paper; I would have stopped by McDonald's on my way to work to calm myself with two sausage biscuits, hash browns, and a large coke. If I encountered a difficult procedure with a patient, I would simply go into my office, close the door, and eat from the secret stash of M&Ms in my desk drawer, or Snickers from under the sink in my private bathroom, or Kit-Kats from my purse. On the way home from work, I frequently buffered my feelings with fast food snacks before going home to have supper with my family. I functioned quite well as long as I was not far from food.

I was unaware that food had become my primary way of soothing stress. Now, my new self-awareness sent me into a spiral of self-loathing. I felt demoralized and frightened to suddenly understand how "sick" I was. Cut off from my fix of a steady supply of food, I was forced to face myself. No longer just concerned about my physical condition, I was now thinking of my emotional and mental health as well.

I gathered myself together the best I could and headed to the dining room. Lunch made me feel a little better—which made me feel even worse. *You're using food even here, the very place you're supposed to be learning to eat appropriately. You're sick, worthless.* And so the waves rose again.

After lunch, I met with Patricia, the counselor I'd been assigned, and the venom just poured out, all aimed at myself. She let me talk and cry until exhaustion stopped me. Finally I asked the question that I'd been trying to drown out. "What's wrong with me? Normal people don't get into this state over a lost piece of paper. People like you and Glenn would just let it go. What's wrong with me?" My husband Glenn, always steady, never seemed to let little things bother him.

After waiting patiently to be sure I'd finished my thought, she stood and walked to her desk across the room, retrieving a new box of Kleenex. I took several from the fresh box and blew my nose. Still she waited patiently as I sat slumped and miserable.

Finally she spoke quietly and reassuringly, but her words surprised me. "You're right, Hilda. While 'normal' people do get upset over little things sometimes, they get over it more quickly because they have a skill that you never learned, never had the opportunity to learn."

I sat up a little straighter. She had my full attention.

She slowly ran her fingers through her short curly blonde hair, gently pushing a few strands back from her forehead. After only a few sessions, the gesture was already familiar to me.

"Most people know how to soothe themselves," she said. "Very young children learn the skill while watching their parents. When parents comfort themselves and their child, the child learns how to do that for herself. If you grow up in an unsafe and unsupportive home, as you did, you never learn how to do that."

"But you said yesterday in class that an anxiety attack will only last three or four minutes, and that we should learn to ride it out. This one lasted a lot longer than that!"

"Do you remember the graph I showed the class, how anxiety comes down sharply after it peaks?" She picked up a pad and pencil that lay near the empty Kleenex box and re-drew a rough graph, showing a rapid rise to the peak of anxiety followed by a slow drop back to baseline.

I nodded. I'd counted on that drop today, but it hadn't come

She pointed to the rapid rise up to the peak. "This is where people who have good self-soothing skills have a huge advantage. Even before the anxiety peaks, they soothe themselves. It's all done so quickly, and on such an unconscious level, that they don't even notice it. If fact, most of the time, they don't even recognize any anxiety at all."

"But after it peaked, it didn't decline." I pointed to the drop back to baseline.

"Nobody can think very well at that peak, but the brain kicks back in on the downward slope. Unfortunately, as soon as *you* start thinking, that criticizing voice in your head forces you into a new anxiety and a new peak. Over and over again. Each wave may last only a few minutes, but you experience wave after wave. And you were right when you said it probably wouldn't have happened at home because you could use food to calm down. You've learned that food can soothe."

My head was clearer than when I'd come into her office. What Patricia said made sense. I thought about how the morning had gone. The anxiety *had* come in waves and repetitive self-criticism *had* made it worse. And nothing but lunch had helped at all.

"Okay," I began slowly, trying to find the next logical step. "If I didn't learn those self soothing skills as a child, and learned to use food instead, what can I do now? Can I learn those skills *now*, as an adult?"

"Yes and no. You can learn to self-soothe, but not to the degree that a young child does. It will never be instinctive for you like it is for folks who grew up in safe and nurturing surroundings."

I laughed. "So, I'm paying you the big bucks to tell me it's hopeless?"

She smiled as she shook her head. "No, not hopeless, but I'd be misleading you if I told you it'll be easy."

"I'm committed. Tell me where to begin."

"You've already begun," she said. "You didn't squelch the anxiety with food."

"Food? What food? There's no extra food around here." I laughed, but then remembered lunch and felt guilty. "Actually, I did use food," I said. "I used lunch to calm myself down a little."

"We all use food for comfort sometimes, and there's nothing wrong with that. But Hilda, please give yourself some credit. You have a car. There's a Burger King, a Wendy's, and a McDonald's within a few blocks. Not to mention the bakery down the street. You could've easily eaten your way out of this anxiety. Many people who come here do just that. You were willing to feel the pain. And the fact that you understand how you used food for comfort in the past is a huge first step. Now congratulate yourself for the incredible work you've done today. And don't let that nasty inner critic undermine you."

I hesitated. "I'll try," I said slowly, suspecting the task would be harder than it appeared. "Tell me where to go from here."

"You have two tasks. First, reduce the stress in your life so you're not constantly living in a state of anxiety. Next, find ways to comfort yourself with something other than food. Some of the classes here will help, but you'll have to just explore what works for you. And make sure you get to the class tomorrow on dealing with your inner critic. Yours is working overtime!"

Patricia glanced at the clock on the table beside me. We both stood and I was surprised, as always, at how tiny she was. Just over five feet, a wisp of a woman, she had a grace about her that made me self-conscious. Standing beside this slim, beautiful, self-confident thirty-something-year-old woman, I felt misshapen, inferior.

I left her office and went to the gym to walk. For the first few minutes, I couldn't shake the shadow of inadequacy I'd felt in Patricia's presence. I wanted to eat, to soothe that disquiet that I was so unaccustomed to allowing myself to feel. But I stayed on the treadmill and resolved to find out more about stress, anxiety, and coping skills, and about how this all related to my eating problem.

Over the next few months, I devoured books on how my unsafe childhood may have affected my ability to cope, and thus contributed to my binge eating. Clearly, not all children growing up in abusive homes become binge eaters, and not all binge eaters come from this sort of home, but there's a strong correlation between the two.[1] I wanted to understand the pathway linking them.

Children, like myself, who grow up in unsafe homes become keenly vigilant to the dangers around them. We scan our world—through sights, sounds, and smells—for signs of danger and take on hypervigilance as a way of life.

In my youth, I wasn't conscious of how vigilant I stayed, but even as a young child, I knew the difference in the sound of Dad's pick-up truck on the gravel driveway when he was drinking and when he wasn't. Straightened sample books in my parents' upholstery shop made my heart quicken; they meant Dad was drinking and Mom had kept busy in the front room, straightening fabric samples, in order to stay out of his way. I lived in a state of readiness. I kept my school books together and near my bedroom door so I could grab them if we had to flee quickly. In the worst of times, I even kept a bag with a change of clothes handy.

These patterns of hypervigilance became deeply engrained. My sisters and I still check exits when we enter a room. We don't sit with our backs to a door or feel comfortable with big men standing behind us. It's not that we get a full-blown anxiety attack or even consciously experience fear. The response of carefully watching our surroundings and being aware of danger is simply always with us.

My youngest sister, Lynni, recently remodeled her bathroom. She put in sparkling new tile on the floor and walls, a vintage fan above, and a huge soaking tub along one wall. Her friends kept asking why she hadn't put in a Jacuzzi during the renovation. Lynni couldn't explain because she really didn't know why; in fact, she would have *liked* a Jacuzzi. One day Deeber, her closest friend since early childhood and the only one of our friends privy to what went on in our home, was at Lynni's when an acquaintance dropped by. Lynni showed off her newly remodeled bath, and sure enough, the question of the Jacuzzi came up. "I don't know," Lynni answered vaguely. "I just didn't think about it at the time, I guess."

After the acquaintance left, Deeber said, "Lynni, you *do* know why you didn't put in a Jacuzzi."

"Why?" Lynni asked, puzzled.

"Just think about it," Deeber said.

Lynni thought for a minute and finally shook her head. "No, I really don't know why."

"It's too loud. You wouldn't be able to hear your dad coming."

That hypervigilance has stayed with us even though circumstances are totally changed and the conscious fear is gone. Dad's been dead for years and Lynni's not afraid in her home, but somewhere deep in her psyche, far removed from mere thought, remains the need to clearly hear everything in order to stay safe.

There is a primitive part of our brain, called the amygdala, which is at least partially responsible for these lasting reactions to danger. The amygdala is first in line for information coming from our various senses. It's a sort of triage station where information is quickly assessed. If the information requires normal thought, the amygdala sends it on to the more advanced thinking part of the brain, where deliberate and measured decisions are made. But if the amygdala senses an emergency that demands *immediate* action, it doesn't take the time to send a transmission to the thinking brain. It simply reacts.[2]

Most of us have faced an emergency situation where we just reacted without thinking. Perhaps we saw a semi-truck and slammed on the brakes or swerved before we even processed the fact that we saw the truck in the first place. Afterward, we might have said, "I just acted. I couldn't seem to think." And we were right—we literally could not think. At that moment, we were functioning in our amygdala where thought isn't possible.

This amygdala, with its unique ability to bypass thought, was what kept humans alive thousands of years ago when we were threatened by bears and tigers, and it's what keeps us alive in an immediate crisis today. Unfortunately, there are some problems with this handy little amygdala.

For one thing, it's very sensitive to continued use. The more our brains route information through it, the more easily triggered these neural pathways become. The younger we are, the quicker the pathways form, and the stronger and deeper the grooves.[3] As a child, when I was constantly vigilant in my home, rarely relaxing, the grooves of my amygdala were changing, becoming virtual ruts. I was being programmed to function in crisis mode, to act from the amygdala.

Another problem with the amygdala is that it isn't very discriminating. When even one key element is present from a past danger, the amygdala may call it a match. And because it responds so rapidly, it often reacts to incomplete, even inaccurate, information.[4] A real threat and a perceived threat often look the same to this primitive brain.

Because I grew up hypervigilant to danger, I associate many sights, sounds, and smells with an emergency situation. In fact, my amygdala has a hair-trigger. It readies me for action quickly and often, leaving me in a state of anxiety much of the time. One way it does this is through the release of the stress hormone, cortisol. Cortisol is an interesting hormone. It results in the laying down of visceral fat in the abdominal area.

Interestingly, this fat is more metabolically active than fat just under the skin, and can be more quickly converted to energy for a fight-or-flight situation.[5]

Since I didn't learn to self-soothe, I couldn't hush even little moments of stress. Bombarded with these feelings of anxiety, I often turned to my easily accessible and sure means of comfort: I ate. In fact, if I could trace the source of my cravings, I would probably find some cue in the environment to which my amygdala reacted. It only takes a tiny fragment of some memory to trigger this whole system. And food worked for me. At least temporarily. In the moment, food (especially sweet, fatty foods since they have the power to block the release of some stress hormones[6]) calmed me and I felt better, but the residue of shame only led to more stress and more eating. And on and on, until I became a chronic binger with major health issues.

In addition to this hypervigilance, however, there was an added emotional factor in place in my family, as there is in so many families like ours. Mom, beaten down decade after decade, both literally and figuratively, felt as powerless as we did. She did not, and most likely could not, act on our behalf.

Mom didn't gather us up that Christmas to comfort and reassure us. She didn't stroke our hair or kiss our cheeks or in any way sooth our wounded spirits. She didn't take us in her arms and run, screaming, out of that mad house. We just went on pretending that everything was normal, occasionally leaving for the safety of an aunt's house, but always returning.

At our mother's knee, we learned the deadliest of skills. Silence. We were silent about our home life with everyone. Silent with our friends and neighbors. Silent with each other. But worst of all, we were silent about the truth within ourselves. I was filled with an unacknowledged self-loathing because I hated my dad. Filled with an unexpressed shame when I placed toys at the top of the stairs after everyone had gone to bed, hoping Dad would trip and fall. Filled with a dreadful anxiety that he would actually fall. Then filled with both an unsatisfying relief and unspeakable fury when he didn't. I was also filled with a private dark envy for the family across the alley whose drunken father committed suicide after years of abuse to his family. Just the month before he killed himself, he threw one of his children down the stairs and broke the child's arm. Life in our housing project was not pretty, but the silence we maintained was the most damaging part of all.

Looking back, it seems incredible that each of us chose to live in our own separate, silent worlds. My sisters and I have always been close, so it's hard for us to understand why we never talked to one another about what was going on, or about what we were feeling. I suppose keeping the silence helped us keep our world "normal." We wanted above all else to be normal, to be like our friends and schoolmates. If we'd spoken of it, the horror and the craziness of it might have spilled out of the box in which we kept it safely locked away. The silent, pretend world in which we each lived protected us from directly facing a life we were incapable of understanding or dealing with in any constructive way.

The silence we learned to live with during those years may have kept us all feeling safe and sane at the time, but it also kept us ill for many years. For the first five decades of my life, I hid the truth of my childhood and the truth of how I used binge eating to cope with the pain of that abuse. And because of that silence, I stayed locked in shame, unable to get help for my problem.

Mom neither soothed us, nor acknowledged that we needed to be soothed. According to Patricia, self-soothing is the earliest, most primal, and probably most essential of all coping skills. Only in a safe and nurturing environment, where the need to be comforted is acknowledged, can it be learned.

In an ideal home and in an ideal world, as a baby is nursed at her mother's breast and comforted by the warm milk that satisfies her hunger, she watches her mother's smiling face, and connects to the sweet smell of her mother's body. She hears her calming voice, and is comforted by her loving touch. All the senses are stimulated and bundled together in this safe environment, and the child is soothed.

If this child, at four, is frightened by the "boogie man" in her room at bedtime, she runs screaming to her father who immediately takes her in his arms. Kissing her forehead, he speaks to her in a calm soothing voice and sings a favorite lullaby. Returning with her to the bedroom, he shows the child that the "boogie man" was only a shadow on the wall. This scenario may happen more than once, but the child eventually convinces herself it is indeed only a shadow. She learns to soothe herself, and learns that her home is a safe place in which to grow up.[7]

Compare this nurtured child to the child who grows up neither safe nor happy. She, too, may be held by her well-meaning mother who feeds her with comforting food. But what else does this child see and experience? Anger, sadness, and fear are telegraphed to the child through her mother's eyes, her touch, her voice, and even her smell. Mother and father yell, and siblings cry. As she grows up, this young child may be physically, even sexually, abused. In *her* home, the shadows on the wall are real.

As this young girl grows, she may take on any number of destructive coping skills. For example, she may become hostile and begin acting out. She may display infantile behavior and refuse to "grow up." The child may become depressed and withdrawn. As she enters adolescence, she may become promiscuous in order to get the attention and comfort she needs. She may turn to alcohol or drugs or gambling or shoplifting. The list is almost endless.

Even if a child is not held and snuggled and sung to when she's fed, the act of eating and the food in her belly gives her pleasure and nourishment. Eating is one of the earliest and most consistent comforts we experience, and one that stays with us long after we reach adulthood. It is not that the neglected or abused person has *no* means of comfort other than food, or that every abused child will turn to food for comfort. Most of us will find at least some comfort in other areas of our life, but for children growing up in an unsafe environment the range of choices is far more limited and the key ability to self-soothe is greatly dampened.

I don't know when I first began to binge on food for comfort, but I do have an early memory of hiding under the kitchen table with Mom's pink-and-white-flowered sugar bowl and a loaf of bread. I must have been about four. Mom and Dad were in the next room. He was yelling, she was crying. I poured sugar on the soft white bread, folded it, and pinched the edges to seal in the sugar, and secretly ate sugar sandwiches one after the other.

For years, I'd known that I used food to get through major stresses. What I hadn't realized, however, until that day I sat weeping in a back hall at Duke, was that I used food, sometimes on an hourly basis, just to get through the smallest of upsets. For most of us in America, food is immediately available, and it comforts and soothes in the most primal way possible. But as food became my *primary* means of comfort, it severely limited my emotional growth and well-being, and threatened my physical health.

Through all the years that I suffered the shame and guilt of binge eating, I had no way of knowing that trauma in my childhood had had such an impact. I didn't know that it had caused not only psychological problems, but actual physical changes in my body. Changes that predisposed me to cravings and bingeing. Armed with this new information, I could finally believe that my bingeing was not the result of a character flaw. I could release the shame associated with binge eating. It may have been stress that triggered the binges, but it was the subsequent shame of the binge that so often circled me back to more stress and more bingeing. I could finally begin to see a way to break that cycle.

My unsafe childhood rendered me chronically stressed, emotionally crippled, and biologically prone to bingeing. I would soon learn, however, that the roots of my binge behavior was far more complicated than simply these early childhood problems.

Chapter Three

Chasing an Illusion: The Chronic Dieter

1964

My stomach growled. I glanced to either side. No one seemed to notice. Most of the class continued to focus on our English Lit teacher, while several stared out the window. We pretended to listen to Miss Davis as she rambled on about the historic background of *Great Expectations*. We all wanted the class to be over. Clearly, this was going to be a long year for the Butler High senior class of 1965.

My stomach growled again. I felt clammy and nauseous and wished I could borrow the flat fan that Miss Davis furiously waved in front of her flushed face. The Jesus figure blurred as it swished back and forth. The five-inch stick handle of the fan remained stiff even in her sweaty palm. No matter how desperately she fanned, she couldn't seem to cool herself.

Classrooms in Alabama in early fall were still hot and muggy, and Miss Davis seemed to suffer more than most. Every day, we looked forward to her turning a bright red, sweating profusely, and wilting before our very eyes. What Mom called change-of-life hot flashes, I guess. Miss Davis' thinning hair glistened as her scalp sweated. She never moved far from her desk or from her First Baptist Church fan. If that fan failed her, I think she might have ignited, or even exploded. The image of splotched skin, stringy wet hair, and fragments of Jesus scattered all over the room increased my queasiness.

The distinct metallic aftertaste of my breakfast Tab added to my discomfort. Now I was sorry I hadn't eaten a little something as well. Usually one Tab for breakfast and another for lunch would hold me, but I'd skipped last night's supper too. Thank goodness for one-calorie Tab! I never dreamed a *diet* soda was even possible, but Coke had come out with Tab last year and now it was all the rage. Since we had no vending machines in our school, I stocked cans of warm Tab in my locker, along with the popular Metracal shakes guaranteed to make me thin.

As a young girl, I'd considered myself pudgy, even though my pictures didn't seem to show it. By age ten, I was taller, heavier, and more developed than any of my classmates. My adolescent years had brought their own special misery. In those years, my developing breasts and hips made me fair game for the boys' teasing. Barry was the worst.

"Is that a camel hair sweater you're wearing?" he'd once asked me loudly as he turned to face me on the crowded school bus. Since my house was at the end of the bus line, I always had to stand. Barry always stood close, but today he was a little too close.

"No," I said, wedging my books between us and bracing myself against the nearest seat as the school bus doors slammed shut. The bus jerked forward.

He nudged pimpled-faced Benny next to him. "Well, then what are those two humps?"

My face flashed red. I fought back tears. All the boys laughed. I could feel their eyes staring at my jiggling breasts as the bus jerked and rumbled on.

In junior high and high school, I was not one of the "popular" girls. Not like the pretty ones, the cheerleaders, and the Dixie Debs majorettes. I looked in the mirror and saw why. I didn't care what my sisters said, or what the scales showed, the mirror didn't lie. I'd started dieting in the sixth grade and had been counting calories ever since, but no matter what I did or what the scales showed, the mirror told me I was growing fatter and fatter. Dene said I was crazy, but I knew what I saw.

I was a well-liked leader, though, active in numerous clubs, and an officer in several. Always the responsible straight-A student, if you wanted a hard-working, get-it-done person to head your committee, I was your girl. I'd been elected the senior girl most-likely-to-succeed, and had always assumed I was socially ok, if not "popular."

The bell finally released us from Miss Davis' English class. I rushed into the hall and made a beeline for my locker, while most of my classmates headed to the lunchroom. A little shaky, I was saved by a Tab and one last Ayds candy cube. Ayds Diet Supplements could usually get me through the worst of my hunger pangs. Visions of cheeseburgers, onion rings, and vanilla malts tormented me, but I banished them from my thoughts as I skipped lunch and made my way to the Science Club meeting. I focused on the friends I would see there instead of my growing hunger.

The main agenda for the Science Club meeting that day was to start the process of picking a club Sweetheart to represent us in the Homecoming parade. Marilyn and Peg were sure to be nominated, and it would be hard to know who among my friends to vote for when voting day came.

The nominations opened. "Marilyn, I nominate Marilyn" someone said. Then I heard Mike: "I nominate Hilda."

Oh, my God! How can he do such a thing?

I thought I heard snickering.

If it had been anybody else but Mike, I would have thought they were being cruel. Like nominating the fattest girl in school to the homecoming court as a mean joke. But not Mike. Mike was one of the dearest friends I'd had since the fifth grade and there was not an unkind bone in his body. He had no idea how humiliating this was. I didn't hear anything else that happened in the meeting. I was lost in a private panic.

When the bell rang, signaling the end of lunch period, I rushed from the room and headed to the nearest bathroom, remembering taunts from years earlier. *Fatty, fatty, two-by-four. Can't get through the bathroom door.*

I hid in one of the stalls and watched as penny loafers passed, rushing to the next class. One pair of shoes remained. When a half-smoked cigarette fell to the concrete floor I figured it was Rita. She was the only girl I knew with enough guts to smoke in the school building. The toe of her unpolished shoe pivoted several times to crush the butt. She walked out and all was quiet. I waited, staring at the putrid green walls, unable to figure a way out of this humiliating situation. But there was nothing, simply nothing, I could do. The thought of being compared to any of the girls nominated was mortifying, but to be compared to Marilyn—slim, beautiful, impeccably-dressed, perfectly-put-together Marilyn—was beyond any humiliation I could imagine. The stiff toilet paper scratched my face as I wiped away tears over and over again.

After the next bell rang, I waited several minutes before leaving the bathroom. I crept down the hall, cut through the girl's locker room, and sneaked out a side door. I'd never cut a class before, much less skipped school, but I'd rather face suspension than see anyone I knew.

The three-mile walk home seemed endless.

S & S Grocery was on my way. Mrs. Savage, the owner, smiled and waved to me from behind the counter. I flushed. She didn't seem to notice that it was the middle of a school day. I headed straight for the sweets' section and quickly gathered up all the Snowballs and M&Ms my week's lunch money would buy. I usually spent my lunch money on whatever extra things I needed: school supplies, underwear, whatever came up. I felt guilty for spending the money, but I couldn't very well tell my parents I skipped lunch every day.

When I reached home, I went straight to my bedroom, fastening the door behind me. No one would be home for hours. I climbed into bed, unwrapped the first pink snowball, and bit into it. Like salve on a sore, the fluffy texture and the sweet taste soothed my hurt. After finishing all the snowballs, I moved on to the M&Ms, eating them by the handful. I put the wrappings into the bag and stuffed it under the edge of my mattress.

I quietly made a vow. *I'll show them. I'll show all of them. I'll lose this extra weight if it kills me!*

I spent my senior year cycling between hunger and bouts of eating sprees, followed by the requisite guilt. I took dieting to a whole new level that year. Looking in the mirror in those days, I saw an unattractive blimp, and thought that was what everybody else saw too. I was wrong. At 5'7" and 128 pounds, I was definitely *not* fat. Looking back at old high school photographs, I'm amazed to see a beautiful, seemingly confident, young woman looking back at me. No one had any idea of how sensitive I was about my body. Or how relieved I was when the votes were counted and Marilyn was elected Science Club sweetheart.

I was not alone in my inability to see myself as others saw me. It's common for young girls to inaccurately judge how their bodies look, and to exaggerate defects. This is especially true for those who develop early. Young girls often see the normal increase in body fat as overweight.

I kept my weight in check during those last few high school years but, because of my distorted body image, I never got to enjoy the beauty of my body. I'm convinced if I'd never dieted, I would probably still have become overweight, but certainly not morbidly obese. I was the typical yo-yo dieter. And I paid the typical price. It would be more than thirty years before I would realize how I damaged my body in those early years and in all the years to come.

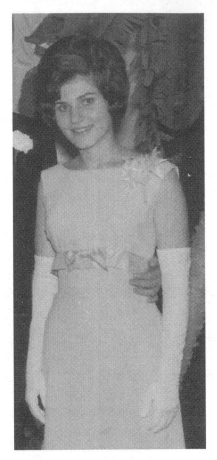

Hilda, senior prom, 1965

1998

Since my early teens, diaries and journals have been a part of my life. As it turns out, that was a stroke of great luck for me. I read somewhere how important journaling could be in uncovering how and why a person overeats. And so, in the spring of 1998, just months after being diagnosed with binge eating disorder, I pulled out all of my old journals and began to analyze them. Through these journals, I uncovered an extreme self-loathing that both saddened and frightened me. A horrifying pattern of dieting and bingeing emerged. Swinging between the two extremes was how I dealt with the agony of self-hatred. In the pages of my journals was written the story of my life. And I didn't like what I saw.

Almost all my entries had to do with my weight and how unhappy I was with my body. I was totally preoccupied with weight and how I looked. Sometimes months would pass with no entries at all, invariably followed by a particularly strong entry about what a failure I was because I'd gained so much weight. Self-loathing was definitely the theme. Reading those entries, I ached for the young girl who wrote:

> *What a worthless failure I am—a weak unmotivated piece of garbage. If other people really knew me, they would despise me.*

After weeks, or sometimes months, of this mental whipping, there inevitably followed a detailed plan of how, *this time*, I would have the will-power to stick to my diet and lose the weight once and for all:

> *OK, I can do this. I can do anything I put my mind to.*
> *I will record every bite I take everyday and will, under no circumstances, eat more than 1000 calories any day. Willpower is all it takes. I can do it!*

Confident each time that I could reach my goal, I diligently tracked, with detailed and meticulous accuracy, my weight and everything I ate. After intense and sustained dieting for several months (during which I typically lost 25 or more pounds), I would describe in the journal some major stress in my life or one of the many nightmares that plagued me, nightmares of being chased and raped or being forced to watch helplessly as my children were tortured and mutilated:

I dreamed a knife nightmare again last night. A man with a knife chased me. I looked back and saw he was gaining. I stumbled. He caught me and pulled me to the ground. I woke up just as he pressed the blade against my throat. I'm so tired...

Then, for several months, silence. No entries at all.

I emerged from these unrecorded periods exhausted, having gained back 30, 40, or sometimes even 50 or 60 pounds. Then an entry would follow where I again expressed self-hatred for having gained back all the weight I'd lost—and then some.

I hate this body! I hate myself for gaining so much weight! What is wrong with me? Why do I keep failing?

I was completely exhausted and lost in guilt, self-pity, and self-flagellation for weeks or months at a time before I emerged once again with a renewed resolve to lose the weight once and for all. And of course, I knew of only one way to regain control: stringent dieting. A battle raged between my body and me, and I resolved to win. I hated my body, and I hated myself for what I saw as a weakness.

And so the cycles continued: months of dieting, followed by months of out-of-control eating, followed by intense self-loathing, then back to rigorous dieting. This destructive pattern went on for decades. With each cycle, I emerged weighing a little more than the time before. With each failure, I learned to hate myself and my body a little more.

I was an intelligent woman, an accomplished, successful adult, always at the top of my class and profession. Why didn't I notice this consistent pattern in my life? But I didn't. Not until I studied my journals years later.

I wept as I read each revealing entry. Wept for the young woman in that journal who hated her body. Wept for the sad woman she had become, and for all the tenderness she had denied herself over the years. As I looked at this fragmented pattern, I realized how much of my life, and my family's life, had floated by because of my obsession with chasing the ideal weight. A great sadness for what I had lost settled over me, and my life slowly began to change.

I am sometimes amazed at the pressure put on women to lose weight, both from within ourselves and from our society. America is a culture obsessed with thinness, a culture at war with our own bodies. While the average American woman is 5'4" and weighs 166 pounds,[1] the average American model is 5'10" and weighs only 107 pounds.[2]

If I felt pressured in high school to reach the ideal size ten or twelve advertised by Tab and Ayds and Metracal, I can only imagine what today's young girl must feel. Size *zero* dresses are at the front of fashion boutiques; the tens and twelves, if carried at all, are hidden in the back of the store.

In the 2014 Miss USA contest, Miss Indiana made headlines because she wasn't as thin as her competition. She was praised for being a "normal" size.[3] Ironically, at a size *four*, she was hardly normal! In 1960, when I was in junior high, the average Miss America contestant wore a size ten; in 2000, she wore a size two;[4] today, sizes double- and triple-zero are not uncommon for the contestants. How can a young woman ever live up to that impossibly thin ideal? And what price will her young body and psyche pay for trying?

While males certainly feel the pressure to maintain a certain body image, females are still more at risk in our culture of thinness because we are taught that our value lies in our physical *appearance* while men are raised to believe that their *abilities* and *achievements* give them worth. Even when they are infants, we speak to girls and boys differently: the girl is "such a pretty little thing" while the boy is "a big, strong fellow."

The pursuit of an ideal, reachable by only a miniscule few and at a huge cost to their health, has led to severe body dissatisfaction for almost every American woman. So what do we do? We diet. By the millions, we diet. Practically every woman, and the majority of young girls, in this country are dieting. In 2000, 50% of nine-year old girls, 80% of middle school girls, and over 90% of senior high school girls dieted regularly.[5] And the trend is getting worse. A recent study showed that 33% of five-year-olds are on some sort of dietary restrictions.[6] Dieting in this country is a multi-million dollar enterprise. This industry has a vested financial interest in keeping the American woman dissatisfied with her body and hungry—always hungry—for ways to change it.

After examining the research, I became convinced that overly restrictive diets simply do not work. Moreover, I was astounded to learn that dieters not only regain the weight they lose, but in the process often turn to bingeing. In fact, dieting has been indicted as the most immediate trigger for binge eating.[7]

Our bodies will not let us hold our breath until we die; we will pass out and begin breathing again. Nor will our bodies allow us to purposely starve to death (except with anorexia). A post-diet bingeing episode is the equivalent of passing out after holding our breath. Our bodies simply refuse to let us starve. When the body gets less food than it needs, it switches to survival mode, turning down our metabolism in order to hang on to every little calorie. Likewise, the mind hits the survival button and turns all its attention to one purpose: find food, find lots of it, and find it fast.

Ironically, I didn't appreciate my body for saving me each time I "failed" and I certainly didn't blame the unrealistic diet I'd escaped for my failure. Instead, I hated my body for "betraying" me and I berated myself for failing (yet again). With that sense of failure came depression, anxiety, and lowered self-esteem. Separately, both hunger and negative feelings could trigger a binge for me; when they occurred together, which was frequently the case since I dieted so much, a binge episode was inevitable. I wasn't alone. According to studies, the most common time for bingeing is when negative emotions pile on top of hunger.[8]

My binge problem kept growing as the effects of my bingeing deepened and broadened with time. In the clutches of the binge, I felt numb, pleasantly isolated from whatever emotion I wanted to escape. Over time, bingeing helped to separate me from *any* and *all* negative feelings for longer and longer periods of time.

I could now see the pattern. My poor body image and generalized self-dissatisfaction had led to dieting in an attempt to make my body more "acceptable." Dieting led to feelings of deprivation, which triggered over-eating and bingeing, setting off even more negative emotions. I would then set new unrealistic goals for weight-loss through yet another diet. And on and on. As I learned that bingeing could temporarily alleviate *any* emotional discontent, I turned to it more and more often. As I continued my quest to learn all I could about binge eating, I discovered that much of the pattern I'd followed was common.[9]

But chronic dieting damaged me more than just emotionally. Severe calorie restriction can, and does, lead to changes in the brain's chemistry that make bingeing more likely to occur. Chronic, highly restrictive dieting can decrease the levels of certain neurochemicals that control impulses.[10] Therefore, when I saw delicious-looking food, my ability to control the impulse to eat was actually reduced *because* I dieted. Dieting can also dampen the innate signals of hunger and fullness by decreasing key chemicals in the brain that cause us to feel full and satisfied; over time, these signals may cease to function altogether.[11]

Dieting was a dead-end street for me. Dieting did not get me the body I wanted and, moreover, it led me deeper into bingeing and further away from my goal. Had I continued with highly restrictive diets, I would have gone on bingeing. In order for me to stop bingeing, ending yo-yo dieting was a critical step.

Chapter Four

Driven to Excess: Genetics Matter

1965

D)*on't look at him. Just don't look.* But I couldn't stop myself. I had to look. The tall, broad-shouldered twenty-something-year-old man who sat at the end of the table four seats down from me was the most beautiful human being I'd ever seen. High cheek bones and an angular jaw gave him a strong face. His full lips—not smiling, yet relaxed and corners slightly up-turned—hinted of a confidence I hadn't seen in other young men on campus. He was quiet, didn't enter into chit-chat around the table, but his presence was palpable. His clear, pale blue eyes revealed a gentleness that made me weak. I'd never seen such blue eyes in someone with jet-black hair before.

I stole another glance at him and saw he was looking at me. I quickly picked up my fork and pushed at the roast and green beans on my plate. My cheeks burned. This was so unlike me. Over the years, I'd learned I could meet anyone, talk with anyone, appear at ease in almost any situation. But today, in this man's presence, I couldn't compose myself, couldn't think of anything clever, or even appropriate, to say.

More than a dozen of us sat around the huge table at Hackberry House for Sunday dinner. Hackberry House, a large Victorian home at the edge of the University of Alabama campus, had been converted into a dorm for "academically talented students with limited resources." I was one of twelve students selected to live in this co-op house. We shared the responsibilities of cooking, cleaning, and maintaining the old house in exchange for a drastically reduced housing fee. On Sundays, we could invite guests. This particular Sunday, Linda, one of the seniors in Hackberry House, had invited Butch, her fiancé from Athens State, and his best friend, Glenn, up for the week-end. Glenn had been a blind date for Linda's roommate, Paula, the night before. Word in the house was that Glenn and Paula had not stayed out late.

As soon as dinner was over, I bolted upstairs to my room. I wanted to stay and be charming to this gorgeous man, but I felt if I spoke, only gibberish would come out. If I walked near him, I would stumble and fall. If I looked directly at him, my knees would buckle.

For days, I could think of little else but this tall, handsome, blue-eyed guy who had literally left me speechless. I knew he'd watched me from across the table, and I wondered if I'd ever see or hear from him again. I shouldn't have worried. It turned out that Glenn was as taken with me as I with him. He wasted no time, even though his approach was less than direct. Within a week, he'd arranged with Butch to arrange with Linda to arrange with me for a date to the upcoming Alabama State Fair. We triple-dated with Butch and Linda and another couple they knew. Within a few months, we were engaged. Within a year—after he got his draft notice and we feared he would be sent to Vietnam—we were married.

My sisters and friends ask me how I knew with such certainty that Glenn was *the one*. I had never planned to marry. I'd seen marriage up close and wanted no part of it. I wanted freedom and independence. I wanted choices. I wanted a career. And none of those involved getting married. But when they ask, I tell them of the voice. The little voice over my right shoulder that whispered *Pay attention*. Every time I was in Glenn's presence, I heard that voice: *Pay attention. This is important.*

And I did pay attention. I fell in love with Glenn almost instantly, but I didn't want him to love me—not unless he really loved *me*—and I didn't believe he *could* love me if he knew the real me. This new-found feeling was unlike anything I'd ever felt before and was important enough that I was willing to lose it, and him, if it wasn't genuine. And so I spent hours confessing my short-comings, my sins, my anger, my hatred. I progressed from admitting I stole other kids' milk money In the first grade, to cheating on a test, then purposely failing the test because I felt so guilty.

"I love *you*. I love *all* of you. You're a good person and you don't even know it," he kept saying.

Finally, I broke a silence I'd kept for eighteen years. I shared with him what I'd not shared with a single friend or relative. I told of my family's secrets. Dad's drinking, the fights, the hatred. I told of the toys I placed at the top of the stairs. I told of lying awake at night, praying that he'd trip and die. I put words to shameful thoughts that I could barely admit to myself. "I'm not a good person. A good person doesn't wish their father dead."

Glenn took my face in his hands and kissed my wet eyes and cheeks. "You don't get it. There's nothing you can tell me that will make me *not* love you."

And I believed him. For the first time in my life I believed that I was loved, not for what I appeared to be, not for what I might be, but for what I was at that very moment. And that love has made all the difference.

I knew right away how good Glenn was for me, but it took me a while to understand that I was also good for him, that I was the best thing that ever happened to him. No one could love him the way I could. Even now, after fifty years, we still have a union that astonishes us both. Thank goodness for that little voice that made me pay attention when it mattered the most.

1967

I bent forward to lift my limp, shoulder-length hair and let the cool air from the window unit nearby blow across the back of my neck. July in Alabama is miserable. I repositioned my body on the green and gold paisley sofa, shifting slightly to lie on my right side, and stuffed a flat feather pillow under my protruding belly. This end of the sofa, right next to the window unit in our tiny rental house, had become my favorite spot to perch while pregnant.

With only weeks until my due date, I was huge and almost immobile. Physically, I was ready to have this baby, but a feeling of foreboding kept me anxious. What did I know about caring for a child? A familiar wave of fear and overwhelming responsibility surged through me. Emotionally, I was in no hurry to be responsible for someone else's life. I was content to keep company with a large bowl of chocolate swirl ice cream cradled beside me. At that moment, I would've been happy to stay pregnant forever. The feeling of dread left me as I finished the ice cream. I sat the empty bowl down on the badly worn green shag carpet.

I'd heard about how awful pregnancy could be; how nothing else compared to the nausea of morning sickness, how tired you were all the time, how fat and ugly you felt. But I'd had no morning sickness; I slept better, and longer, than I ever had; and in spite of a tremendous weight gain, I felt good, even beautiful. Big *and* beautiful, that's how I felt. I loved being pregnant!

And the food! Eating was such a pleasure. Food never tasted so good. For the first time in my life, I could eat with abandon and with little guilt. After all, I *was* eating for two. I was surprised at how much I loved dairy: pudding, yogurt, cheese, chocolate milk, ice cream. Anything made with milk, but especially ice cream. I simply couldn't get enough.

The doctors in the OB clinic at the military base where Glenn was stationed were not happy with my weight gain. They said the recommended gain during pregnancy was 20 pounds. I'd already more than tripled that since I learned I was pregnant—and that was in addition to the 35 I'd put on since high school. I kept telling the doctors how good I felt, but they were adamant that I must stop gaining so much weight. Luckily, I rarely saw the same doctor twice. Even when they warned me about my weight gain, I knew no one would really follow up.

Yesterday's visit had been different. Dr. S. didn't mince words.

"Mrs. Lee, your record shows that we've cautioned you many times. You're gaining way too much weight," he said after looking over my chart.

I lay on the table, my legs up in those stirrups. I felt exposed. I hated being so vulnerable. I counted the tiny holes in the beige ceiling tile and tried to ignore the indignity of the exam.

Dr. S. stood up and looked over the sheet that draped my body. He snapped off his gloves and said in his most god like voice, "You're going into the hospital next week if you gain more than a pound. I know we can control your weight there."

He turned to the nurse, "Be sure she's scheduled with me next week. This has gone far enough." He left the room.

My face burned as the nurse helped me off the examining table. I was embarrassed and angry. Dr. S. didn't know me; he only knew what was written in my chart. I hurried out of the clinic, determined to miss my next appointment.

I slowly pushed my body up from the sofa and plodded into the kitchen to fix myself a bite of lunch. I didn't care what they said at the clinic about my weight. I was eating lots of vegetables and protein and all the other things in the booklet I'd received on the first visit. I'd never smoked or indulged in any form of alcohol. Of course I *was* enjoying ice cream, cake, and other sweets, but my blood pressure and labs had stayed stable, and I felt good. I was taking care of my unborn baby. How could that be wrong?

Food helped me push the doctor's threat out of my mind. I would think of other things. After lunch I gathered several books and notebooks and returned to my cool spot near the air conditioner. Dropping the books onto the sofa, I sat back down, and put my swollen feet up on the wobbly coffee table.

Since getting married, I'd lived in a wonderful, safe cocoon. I felt loved, really loved, for the first time in my life. I had no worries, no school, no work. In fact, I had all the time in the world to do whatever I chose. And I'd chosen to work on a genealogy project. I wanted this child to know about its family history. Not my immediate family—that part of my family history was better left safely hidden away. But I wanted to find out about some of our distant ancestors so I could share that heritage with my child..

All my life, I'd heard stories about Sugar Dulin, my great-great-great grandfather on my dad's side, and about his older brother Rice. I assumed "Sugar" and "Rice" were nicknames, but once I started my search for records, I discovered those were their real names, used on official records such as land deeds and wills. I found two different explanations for the origin of their names: one was that rice and sugar were the family's main crops; the other was that their father's favorite food was rice with sugar.

Sugar Dulin made, and lost, several fortunes. He ended up with thousands of acres of land in North Carolina and died a wealthy man. What a shock! All the Dulins I'd known were dirt-poor. I guess the six sons, six daughters, and nearly 100 grandchildren quickly diluted the wealth Sugar had left.

Apparently well-liked, respected, and active in the community, Sugar loved to play. He had a tremendous sense of humor if you could trust what was written about him by his contemporaries. But he, his father, his grandfather, and his sons were also hard-drinking, hard-gambling men, frequently called before the courts for various minor offences. They were charged with libel, disputes over land, and public drunkenness. Even gambling on a Sunday had landed Sugar's grandfather in jail at least once.

As I communicated with various Dulins (by phone and letters), I began to see a pattern.

"Oh, let me tell you about my granddaddy. What a character!" or "I wish you could have met my uncles!" or "I've never met anyone quite like my crazy great-uncle Joe." I heard these same descriptions over and over again. Many Dulins loved to "dance a jig" or were "the life of the party." Dulins apparently "rarely met a stranger" and "would give you the shirt off his back."

But when I asked about these same Dulins' later years, death dates, and how they died, the answer more often than not went something like, "He died the way he lived—drinking." Or, "His liver finally got him." Or "I tried to tell him he shouldn't drive drunk."

Dulins, especially males, were definitely prone to drink. My unborn baby kicked against my ribs and a shiver of fear went through me. What if I had passed on that Dulin gene to my child? Remembering there was still chocolate swirl left, I returned to the kitchen. After finishing my snack directly from the carton, I felt exhausted. I dragged myself back to the sofa and pushed all the books and notes onto the floor. I lay down and propped my head up on the arm of the sofa, my eyes heavy. I drifted off to sleep, wondering about the kind of legacy I would pass on to my child.

1999

I glanced through the window over my kitchen sink. Darkness still blanketed the sky, but I was wide awake and eager for the week-end ahead. Saturday morning, and I wasn't on call. Thank goodness for dental partners. Thoughts of what I would do over the next few days were interrupted by the shrill whistle of the tea kettle. I hurried to remove it from the burner so as not to awaken Glenn. I put a tea bag into my favorite blue mug, poured in the steaming water, and dipped the bag a few times before discarding it. A little Sweet-n-Low, some milk to cool it down, and I was all set.

Holding the mug in both hands to warm them, I sipped the sweet tea as I walked to my study at the far end of the house.

I set the mug on the corner of my large wooden desk and stood on tip-toes to open the blinds over the file cabinet. The sun would be up soon, and I wanted to catch the first morning light. Orderly piles of brightly colored magazines and books lined one wall of my study, and several neatly organized piles of note cards lay in rows on my desk. I smiled with satisfaction. Organization had always been my strong suit.

I thought this week-end might be a good time to begin an article about binge eating for our local newspaper and about what causes it. I'd gathered more than enough information about how childhood trauma and early dieting could lead to severe eating problems. Yet, it felt like something was missing from the mix, like things weren't quite complete. Wanting to "fix" this slightly off-balance feeling is what had awakened me and led me into my office so early this morning. I wanted to look back through my notes before actually starting the writing process; perhaps I'd overlooked something.

Taking a sip of tea, I settled into my comfortable leather chair and thumbed through several stacks of note cards. When I came to those on body image, I slowed down. This was a subject that had engaged my attention many times in the last several months.

I read two or three notes, then came across one that stated that women are inclined to gain weight at puberty, in preparation for their childbearing years. *We all hate that weight gain,* I thought, *but evolution and individual genetics are strong.* And suddenly, there it was—the missing piece of the puzzle, the thing that had been gnawing at me, trying to get my attention. I'd left out genetics! So obvious, and yet I'd conveniently "forgotten" to deal with it. I immediately knew why: I could stop dieting, could even seek counseling for childhood trauma, but what could I do about genetics?

I'm no coward, though, so I decided to engage whatever I could find head-on. I sat down in the floor near the stack of books and journals and started at the beginning, searching specifically for information on how genetics affect obesity, and perhaps even bingeing itself.

I already knew that the capacity to store fat was a critical step in mankind's development. For most of our history, starvation was the primary threat to survival. This threat not only drove us across continents in search of new food supplies, it also caused our bodies to adapt to the lack of regularly available food. In order to survive in times of famine, our ancestors developed the ability to store fat. And this ability was passed on to us. Those who gain weight easily, like me, are actually blessed with the hardiest of human genes; we are best suited to live through food shortages. You might say that survival of the fittest once meant survival of the fattest. But what was once our greatest genetic asset has now become a huge liability. Genetically programmed to deal with scarcity, we now live in a time of abundance.

I thought about how easy it was for me to get convenient, inexpensive, fabulous-tasting, high-fat, high-calorie food anytime of the day or night and almost anywhere I happened to be. So different from our ancestors who often had to struggle for every morsel. In today's world, I needed to travel only a few blocks in any direction to encounter a fast food restaurant, a doughnut or ice cream shop, or a convenience store. I can remember when gas stations sold only gas, oil, and maybe gum; now, they sell all sorts of food. Every hotel, hospital, airport, sports arena—almost any place I could think of—has food in one form or another.

Portion size has grown exponentially in my lifetime. The Cokes my sisters and I shared as children were only six ounces. In 1955, when McDonald's struck a deal with Coca Cola, the only size drink served there was seven ounces. By the 1990s 42 ounces was the typical large size in most fast food places. A quick look at Seven-Eleven's soft drink history tells the story of super-sizing in America: it went from the Big Gulp (32 ounces) in 1986 to Super Big Gulp (44 ounces), Double Gulp (64 ounces), the X-Treme Gulp (52 ounces), and finally, in 2006, to the Team Gulp (at a whopping *128* ounce)![1]

In the late '50s, when I ate my first fast food hamburger, it was one ounce, typical at the time; now a regular hamburger is six ounces and the larger ones are twelve.[2] Hardee's Monster Thickburger has 1420 calories. And have you seen the video clip about the Las Vegas restaurant that serves an 8000 calorie cheeseburger?[3] The names of fast food products tell the story of increased portion size: Biggie Fries, Big Grab, Whopper, Big Mac, The Beast. Taco Bell's "Fourth Meal," which is touted as the late night meal between dinner and breakfast, normalizes eating to excess, day or night.

And they make it so easy for us to over-consume! How can we resist the second apple pie at McDonald's when we can often get two for a dollar, or pay 89 cents for one? Or a second dozen Krispy Kreme doughnuts for only a dollar more?

No wonder nearly 70% of Americans are either overweight or obese.[4] There's been a 370% increase in the number of people who are morbidly obese in this country since 1970.[5] Our genetics of famine is not serving us so well in this environment of feast.

Genetics of famine in an environment of feast. I jotted down the catchy phrase and moved on.

Males and females have different patterns of weight gain during their adolescent years and different physiological eating demands on their bodies. A young boy begins to crave protein at puberty in order to built muscles; he has a net weight gain due to these muscles, but actually *loses* body fat during those years. A budding young girl, on the other hand, develops strong cravings for fats and carbohydrates in order to quickly and efficiently store fat; her percentage of body fat goes up during her adolescent years.

The reason for these differences is quite simple: for thousands of years the goal of humans was to live long enough to produce a child and have that child live long enough to also reproduce. The young girl's body prepared her for childbearing. She needed extra stored calories in order to support a pregnancy, feed the nursing baby, and survive while she cared for the young child. The young man needed to develop strong muscles in order to hunt and kill the wild boar for himself and his dependant family.

I didn't just *desire* to eat during my early teens. Like all young women, I felt a strong physiological *demand* to eat. This powerful protective mechanism forced me to put on fat in order to insure fertility and the survival of a potential child.

My large weight gain during pregnancy was, to a great extent, my body's way of helping me protect my baby. Because I'd been eating so poorly all through high school, my body was ill-prepared for a healthy pregnancy. My high school diet of Tabs, toast, and Twinkies just wasn't good enough to support a growing baby. So my body did what was needed to protect my child: it *demanded* that I eat. This is not to deny the fact that I also ate to soothe my emotions during pregnancy. I was terrified of the responsibility of motherhood.

I was glad to be able to hide behind those maternity clothes, "hatching jackets" as we called them in the '60s. What I hatched was a healthy seven pound, twelve ounce baby boy, and a blimp of a young mother!

As I kept digging into the literature, I discovered that genetics not only has a role in weight and obesity in general, but also affects the actual *behavior of bingeing itself*. I knew that eating disorders in general tended to run in families,[6] but I'd never considered the possibility that a behavior seemingly so grounded in emotions could be influenced by my genetic make-up. Twin studies, however, made me reassess my thinking. One study of binge eating, for example, showed that the correlation for binge eating is three times stronger between identical twins than between fraternal twins.[7] Several other studies have pointed to bingeing as about half heredity and half environmentally induced.[8]

Obesity experts have long suspected that some people might have a genetic alteration in certain genes that control satiety and fullness. This area of research had tantalized scientists for decades, but the answers had to wait until the science of gene mapping could advance. And advance it did.

In March of 2003, *The New England Journal of Medicine* published a study that examined the genetic make-up of over 1000 extremely obese people. They found that one in twenty of them actually had a specific gene mutation.[9] These people are *missing* certain neurochemical receptors that control satiety, so they literally never get the signal that they are full and should stop eating. These neurochemical receptors, by the way, are the same ones that can be altered with chronic dieting. The most compelling finding of the study, though, was that *every person* with the mutated gene reported binge eating regularly, while only 14% of equally obese subjects (but who did *not* have the mutated gene) reported binge eating.[10] The mutated gene, then, is linked directly to binge eating behavior itself and not just to extreme levels of obesity. The study concluded that the behavior of binge eating is highly heritable.[11]

The vast majority of us, however, have *not* inherited the mutated gene for severe bingeing, and we may or may not have some inherited *tendency* to binge. A full 95% of the obese subjects in the study did not have the mutated gene for obesity, yet were equally as obese as those who did. Just the normal human genetic make-up is enough to make us fat when it meets up with today's environmental forces.

Genetically programmed to deal with scarcity, we now live in a time of abundance. In the past, the genetic tendency to store excess fat was not fully expressed in most people. Food was not readily available and much physical labor was required to just catch, grow, and prepare food. But that has drastically changed, at least in our western culture. Our genes may determine our potential, but it is the environment that allows that potential to be realized. Well-known obesity expert George Bray said it best: "Genes load the gun, but environment pulls the trigger."[12]

Leaning back in my desk chair, I clasped my hands behind my head and sighed. I had mixed feelings. The scientist in me was pleased because I'd found what I was looking for: I'd found evidence pointing to a strong link between genetics, obesity, and even binge eating. But as a person who wanted and needed to be in control, I felt discouraged. I didn't know what to do with all this information. If the genetic role was so strong, did I really have any chance to control my binges?

My chest tightened. My heart rate went up. My breathing became short and shallow. I felt the anxiety and recognized the signs of an oncoming binge, but felt powerless to stop it.

I knew I was making progress in my efforts to stop bingeing. About a year had passed since I'd started my journey back to health and I was bingeing far less often and less severely. And the weight was also dropping—I'd already lost 60 pounds. But I'd lost 60 pounds on many occasions in the past. What if this was just another cycle? I tried to push the doubt and the mounting feeling of hopelessness away, but I could feel myself entering a spiral, could hear the beast calling my name. I resisted, but the siren song was strong and sweet.

By now, it was mid-morning and Glenn was in the yard doing some clean-up. From everything I'd learned, I knew I should join him there, should get active, divert my mind from this growing desire to eat. I should go for a walk. Read a book. Take a shower. Cry. Scream. Anything but what I knew I was about to do. But nothing in me wanted any part of the positive things I'd learned. And so I did what I'd done on so many occasions before: I hurried to the kitchen and calmed myself with food.

Two light sandwiches, two yogurts, and a full bag of baked chips later, I began to relax and talk myself down. Glenn and I went for a walk, then I took a long shower.

I didn't return to my study that day. In fact, I left the mess just as it was, with books open, notes scattered. I spent the rest of that Saturday taking care of myself and talking myself out of a major binge.

Sunday morning came and I returned to the research. Perhaps I'd find something positive, or at least a way to put a positive spin on things so I could escape from the pit into which I was slipping.

Trying to find a thread to follow, I went back through the indexes of several books. Ironically, since I was so down, I came across the fact that there is a strong correlation between binge eating and depression. In fact, half the people diagnosed with binge eating disorder are depressed or have been depressed in the past.[13] One study showed that people with binge eating disorder are at an increased risk for depression and anxiety, while those who are equally obese but who do not binge are not at greater risk.[14] Does depression cause binge eating, binge eating cause depression, or is the correlation genetic in nature? There was certainly no way I could sort it out in my own life. The studies, however, seem to suggest that there are shared genetic factors that might predispose some people to both depression and binge eating.[15] In fact, there is a strong correlation between binge eating disorder and all sorts of psychological issues such as depression, anxiety, PTSD, bipolar, and increased suicide risk.[16]

What really got my attention, however, were studies suggesting a strong correlation between binge eating and alcoholism and other substance abuse. Not only is the binge eater more likely to abuse alcohol and drugs (50% of those with eating disorders engage in substance abuse compared with 9% of the general population[17]), but *family members* of the binge eater are three to four times more likely to have an abuse problem than people who have no relatives with binge issues.[18] This observation, of course, brought to mind the age-old argument concerning environment versus genetics. In my own family, for example, was my brother's alcohol addiction, a sister's past drug problems, and my own binge eating the result of us all growing up under the same roof, with the same stresses, or was a genetic factor at work? Since studies show that the correlation holds true even when the relatives are not in the same household—distant-living uncles, grandparents, and nephews are often affected—a true genetic influence must be at work.[19]

Exactly how binge eating and substance abuse are connected is unclear, but the literature seems to point to the idea that binge eating and substance abuse may simply be different responses to the general genetic trait of *impulsivity*. Studies show, for example, that those who binge, as well as their families, tend to be impulsive, unrestrained, stimulus-seeking people who go after the exciting, novel, intense experience.[20] Those traits would probably mean they tend to be adventurous entrepreneurial risk-takers in business as well as play. Recent studies point to a connection between binge eating and other impulsive disorders such as ADHD.[21] In fact, brain scans of patients with ADHD and BED show similar imaging.[22] I couldn't help but think of the lifestyle of Sugar and Rice and so many of their impulsive descendants right down to me and my siblings.

This whole idea of impulsivity linking various behaviors reminded me of a man I once met. He had given up his credit cards because he sometimes shopped compulsively. He only did so, however, subsequent to binge eating. He said when he binged on food and he got to the point where his stomach could no longer hold another bite, he would often turn to binge shopping on late night TV in an attempt to satisfy the same urge that had brought on his binge eating. This behavior was taking a toll on the family's finances, so he and his wife decided he should simply not have credit cards.

If binge eaters tend to be impulsive risk-takers, what about their opposites: restricting anorexics? I found studies that show that patients with anorexia, and their families, are highly *averse* to risk-taking and commonly show great emotional control, follow the rules, and are quite conscientious.[23] Interesting contrast.

I thought about my own family: my parents, siblings, children, and more distant relatives. Rarely do you find a quiet introvert in the group. Never accused of being lukewarm, we are mostly verbal, very impulsive, and generally unrestrained. My father, of course, was an alcoholic. One of my half brothers died from alcoholism-related health issues in his forties. Another half-brother died in the Korean War after joining the Army and becoming a paratrooper at barely seventeen. Two of my siblings are recovering alcoholics, one has a history of drug abuse and dangerous sexual encounters, and we all have eating problems to one degree or another. Depression, anxiety, ADHD, even bipolar disorder plague my family.

I took a deep breath, turned away from these destructive traits, and tried to think of our family's more constructive ones. We love competition and are avid game-players. We have a fair number of creative individuals in our midst. There's no doubt that many of us are willing to take risks and are entrepreneurial by nature, as evidenced by my dad's upholstery shop (and the many other businesses he tried before succeeding at that one), one sister's drapery business, another's tax service, my own dental practice.

Suddenly, and for no apparent reason, I remembered an obscure study I'd recently come across. I wasn't sure how, but it seemed relevant to my present train of thought. I retrieved the green folder on the far side of the desk and shuffled through several stapled sheets before I located it.

The investigation, small and certainly not conclusive, had intrigued me for weeks. That's why the folder had remained on my desk and not filed away. In the study, normal-weight and obese individuals were asked to sit alone in a room until called. The room was furnished with a chair, a table, a lamp, and a painting on the wall. Each subject was left in the room the same amount of time and was then taken to another room where each was asked to describe the first waiting room (they had not been told that they would be asked to describe the room or that this was actually the study itself). The normal-weight individuals listed, without embellishments, the objects in the room: a chair, a table, etc. The obese individuals, on the other hand, gave a much more detailed description of the room: an oak chair upholstered in forest green leather, a brass lamp with a beige textured shade, a painting of a mountain scene, and so on.[24]

One interpretation of this study is that obese individuals may be more sensitive to environmental cues than their thinner counterparts. This would make them more likely to respond to the sight of a Big Mac, or to the smell of fresh cinnamon buns in the mall, or hot popcorn in the movie theater. Brain scans do, in fact, demonstrate that people with binge eating disorder have a heightened sensitivity in the reward centers of their brains compared to the brains of non-bingeing individuals.[25]

But there was something else about that study, something that kept pulling at me, and wouldn't let go. Some part of me wanted to connect this characteristic of being hyper-aware of the environment with the trait of being an impulsive risk-taker.

I imagined an early tribal community. At the edge of the village were the more adventurous, risk-taking individuals. They were the ones willing, and often eager, to seek out the distant edges of the forests in order to find new food supplies, or to do battle with neighboring tribes for control of natural resources. Many courageous risk-takers ventured out, but only a few returned safely. Who survived to lead their kin to better hunting grounds? It had to be the ones with a heightened sense of vigilance, the ones who could quickly recognize and react to danger.

It seems safe to assume, then, that people (like many in my family) who inherit an impulsive nature are probably also more in touch with cues from their environment. It took both the stimulus-seeking impulsiveness to explore *and* the hypervigilance to ensure survival; survival for the individual as well as for the human species. We are indebted to those ancestors. Even today, our small businesses and large companies may be populated with descendants of those individuals. The *combination* of the impulsive, stimulus-seeking, risk-taking trait with the characteristic of being in tune with the surrounding environment was indeed a blessing for mankind.

But, as with so many blessings, I knew there was a curse attached. The young tribesman who had both traits was well suited for the adventure of stepping into the unknown, but not so suited for ordinary village life. I imagine that the descendants of that young tribesman struggle with the challenge of harnessing those traits in the modern world. I suspect many young men who are drawn into the military's elite Special Forces units today may fit the tribesman's profile and, as we so often see, may not be cut out for civilian life. We want our returning heroes to turn off the very characteristics that keep them alive and willing to fight our battles.

Perhaps the curse goes beyond the misfit soldier or the western frontiersman who couldn't settle down in the town he helped to tame. Perhaps the curse of the pairing of these ancient traits shows up in alcoholics, drug addicts, shoplifters, compulsive gamblers. And binge eaters. Treatment centers and hospitals, courtrooms and prisons may be filled with the blessing/curse run amuck.

It was only a theory, but my mind kept whirling around this idea that somehow the merging of the characteristics of impulsiveness and hypervigilance might contribute to some people becoming binge eaters.

I pictured a child who inherits an impulsive risk-taking nature from one or both of her parents. That child is raised in a home where at least one of her parents is probably an impulsive, stimulus-seeking risk-taker. This often means alcohol or drugs or some other destructive habit that will cause unrest in the home. Remember, this child is impulsive by nature, so in order to relieve the intense stress she feels, she may impulsively turn to any number of vices, including binge eating. Additionally, she is more aware of the drugs or the alcohol or the Big Mac to which she may impulsively be drawn. She is, then, in *triple* jeopardy: her impulsive nature, her awareness of cues around her, and the home into which she is likely to be born all conspire to make her a binge eater, or worse.

I ran both my hands through my short hair and rapidly scratched my head, a gesture I'd seen my mom do often. I felt trapped by my own genetics. I remembered a Dulin I'd met the year before. His father had seven brothers, six of whom had already died of alcohol-related problems. The man was extremely proud of the businesses that his great-uncles had built from the ground up, but was angry at them for being so destructive with alcohol. But those brothers, like our young tribesman, could not readily shut down traits when it would have been healthier and safer to do so. No, they come in a package deal.

There's no question that I have these paired traits. They have been my blessing and my curse. They're the genetics that delivered me into the toxic home into which I was born, but they're also the traits that kept me alive in that home. I was super-aware of the dangers around me, which led to great stress, but even more important, I was able to take fast action when needed, quickly weighing options, because of my ability to read environmental cues.

Likewise, my success in business was due to these same traits. I had a strong drive to succeed, and was willing to risk everything in order to go to dental school, hire the best staff even when cash flow didn't justify it, and construct a new office building at great financial risk. But that willingness to take risks didn't do it alone; I was also strongly aware of those around me and was instinctively in tune with patients and staff. It all came together in an entrepreneurial package that delivered success.

But I couldn't choose to turn those traits off, even though they sometimes controlled me rather than served me. The very traits that helped me be successful in business may be the same ones that made me susceptible to binge eating. If I had the power to strip away what made me binge and, in the process, give up what I consider to be the very essence of me, would I be willing to do so? I love the adventure at the edge of the forest, but I hate the beast I find there. What could I do?

After a long lunch with Glenn and a walk down to the lake to clear my head, I returned to my study to clean up the mess I'd left. I shuffled through loose notes and copies of articles I'd pulled from folders over the last two days, trying to figure out where each one should be filed. But things weren't so clear anymore.

For example, the study on the mutated gene that correlated with binge eating certainly belonged in the new folder I'd made on genetics, but didn't it also belong in some other category? After all, a full 95% of the obese people in the study did *not* have the mutation, yet still became as obese as those who did? Were they simply victims of our environment of feast? If you tracked their life history, would you find unsafe childhood homes? Chronic dieting?

I sat back and looked around at the stacks of note cards, sticky notes, and assorted folders with copies of articles spilling from them. When I'd started my search to understand the causes of binge eating, I'd conveniently and artificially divided them into neat little piles, as if each aspect had nothing to do with the others. But what I saw before me now was a tightly tangled mess that couldn't be teased apart.

In the face of its complexity, I was torn between relief and frustration. I was relieved to find further evidence that my problem was not simply the result of being weak-willed or somehow flawed. By understanding this, I'd been able to release the shame of bingeing, the shame that had crippled me, that had destroyed my spirit little by little. I had begun the real process of healing and could now find constructive solutions.

My frustration, however, was huge. I liked order and clarity, and this was anything but orderly and clear. Plus now I had to reluctantly acknowledge that this beast was much bigger, and the labyrinth in which he held me captive was much more complicated, than I'd imagined. From the beginning, my goal had been to learn all I could about binge eating and its causes so I could destroy this monster that threatened to destroy me. I had been sure that knowledge would equip me to annihilate him.

Once I came face to face with the forces at work against me, however, I feared I would never possess the weapons I needed to conquer that beast and find my way out of the labyrinth. I could never change my personal genetics and the powerful process of evolution. I could never stand completely steadfast in the face of my environment. I could never fully undo the damage done from years of futile dieting. I could never destroy all my personal inner demons. The labyrinth in which I found myself was more twisted, and the monster more ferocious, than I'd ever imagined. The struggle would be hard. I would not be able to overcome the obstacles ahead with any skill I already had. I was going to need more ammunition! I strengthened my resolve, however, and readied myself to face whatever lay ahead.

PART III

STRUGGLING IN THE DARK

Young Theseus was loved by the beautiful goddess Ariadne. She knew him to be brave and strong, but even if he could kill the terrible beast, she feared he might not be able to find his way out of the twisted labyrinth. So, before he departed for the depths of the labyrinth, Ariadne kissed young Theseus and gifted him a ball of golden thread to help guide him back to safety.

Bravely, Theseus donned his shiny armor and unsheathed his mighty sword. Valiantly, he fought the Minotaur at every turn; relentlessly, the Minotaur attacked. Even though Theseus grew weary as he struggled in the shadows, he never gave up.

Chapter Five

Eye of the Binge Storm: Crisis of the Craving

1973

Dr. Eagle's loud voice shattered the three hour silence." Time's up!"

How could time possibly be up? I was nowhere near finished! Glancing quickly through the remaining pages, I realized that I hadn't even completed three-fourths of the exam.

I'd carefully, methodically, but rapidly worked my way through this final exam in a required organic chemistry series. I found no comfort in the fact that, as far as I knew, no one had ever completed one of Dr. Eagle's organic chemistry exams. I reluctantly turned my paper over and glided my slide rule into its black leather case.

So much for getting into dental school.

At twenty-six, I was already "old" by the dental school's Admissions Committee standards. They didn't like my age, or the fact that I'd taken six years to get my Bachelor's degree. Never mind that I'd had two kids since starting college, and traveled with my husband for the three years he was in the Army. What really bothered me, though, was that they didn't seem at all impressed by my nearly perfect GPA in literature, history, and philosophy. I was finding out first-hand how little the humanities and the sciences thought of each other.

The dental school's Admissions Committee had asked to see what I could do with a full-time science load. I was determined to show them I could handle anything they threw at me, so I went back to school full-time, taking all the courses I needed in order to be a viable candidate. I filled the spring semester of 1973 with the last of my dental school prerequisites: Organic Chemistry III, Quantitative Analysis, Physics II, and Calculus. During the previous school year, I'd made A's in all but one of my classes and was confident of an A in all of my courses this semester. All, that is, except this organic chemistry class. Organic chemistry was my nightmare.

Dr. Eagle, my organic chemistry professor, was actually a very good teacher, but he expected an incredible amount of work from his students. Rumor was that his unreasonable demands on students had cost him his position. He was completing his contract that spring semester and had not been invited back to teach in the fall. Over 100 students had started the organic chemistry series in the fall of '72, but at this last final exam for the last organic chemistry course in the series, only *six* of us were left standing—five male premed students and me. Everyone else had either flunked out of Dr. Eagle's class or dropped the course in order to wait to begin a new series with a new professor. But the six of us who'd hung tight had little choice. We were all in the same boat: finish this last class now or wait three semesters for it to be offered again. And waiting was not an option for us since we were all "older" students.

I routinely put in forty hours a week studying for that one class on top of all the time required for my other challenging courses. And my children, Tim and Karen, were at the demanding ages of four and two.

By '73, women may have "come a long way, baby," but not far enough. Only six women, and none with children, had ever been accepted into Alabama's dental school. Female candidates, unequivocally, had to be better than male candidates in order to be considered for the coveted positions.

I knew earning anything less than a B+ in the organic chemistry class would most likely spell rejection.

As we walked out of the exam that day, John, the shortest and one of the brightest in our group, was pale. "I barely got half way through. Did any of you finish?" he asked the group. I was glad to hear that no one else had completed more than I had. Still, I knew there were several problems on the test that I'd never encountered before, so I didn't feel confident about my results.

I simply couldn't go home until I'd soothed myself. Luckily, Peggy Ann's Bakery was only a short drive away.

Forcing myself to breathe normally, I opened the door, walked nonchalantly into the bakery, and stood patiently at the counter. With great deliberation, I counted aloud the number of children who would be at my daughter's *imaginary* birthday party.

"That's ten kids," I said. "So let me have ten of those chocolate cupcakes, five Bear Claws, and five—no, better make that ten—éclairs." I spoke slowly and distinctly, trying to mask the panic I felt inside.

I held my purse tightly against my chest as I waited for the woman behind the glass case to box up my order. Her pink ruffled apron looked silly on her plump middle-aged body. Could she be any slower? She *would* have to be the one who waited on me today. The annoyingly-perky high school blonde would've been better. I remembered wanting to slap the insipid know-it-all smile off her young face, but at least she was fast, unlike ole slow-poke here. I focused hard on the chip in her right front tooth as she slowly—painfully slowly—counted out each cupcake.

I've heard people say they have a fear of some day just standing up and taking their clothes off in church. Maybe right when the congregation begins "Just as I Am." Or of laughing uncontrollably in the most solemn moment of a funeral service, maybe during a moment of silent prayer for our dearly beloved. My fantasy fear was that one day I simply wouldn't be able to stand patiently on the customer's side of the counter while someone in a frilly pink apron methodically counted out the pastries I so desperately needed. Maybe one day I would abandon all social grace, climb over the glass case, and gather up all the soft, gooey confections I could hold. I would simply sit in the floor behind the display case and eat chocolate cake, jelly-filled doughnuts, meringue-topped banana cream pie...

I wanted to scream, "Hurry up!" Instead, I waited for what seemed an eternity for my stack of precious boxes. I paid with cash and dropped my change in the Muscular Dystrophy can by the register. I tried to walk out normally, like a robber might walk down the street with his loot after emptying the cash drawer of some store. As I left, the bell on the door jingled loudly. I glanced back, as if I might be stopped, but no one seemed to notice the sound but me.

At long last, my stash and I were safe in my rusty green VW Bug. I wanted to go home, shut the door, close the curtains, and eat in private, but home was twenty minutes away. So I did the next best thing.

I pulled into the nearby parking lot of a small, anonymous church. The gravel on the driveway crunched as I circled to the back. No one could see me from the road.

Hands shaking, heart pounding, I lifted the first sweet chocolate éclair to my mouth. My teeth glided through the chocolate glaze, into the pastry, and sank into the smooth pudding in the middle. I closed my eyes and sucked the soft custard into my mouth. With each bite, thoughts of the chemistry test and all that rested on it receded a little. By the time I finished all ten éclairs, my worries had faded away. I moved on to the cupcakes, hurriedly but deliberately licking the last traces of the dark chocolate icing from my fingers as I finished the last one. I saved the bland Bear Claws until last so as to cover the smell of chocolate on my breath. I stuffed in the final one. *All finished. Ten éclairs, ten cupcakes, five Bear Claws.*

Calm now, I laid my head back and rested a minute. Then, slowly and methodically, I put all the little wrappers into the big boxes, careful to include the cash receipt (yet another proof of the money I'd wasted over the years from mine and Glenn's already strained college budget). I drove to the nearby Piggly Wiggly, pulled around into the alley, and tossed the evidence of my private orgy into the dumpster with the rest of the trash. I still had plenty of time to drive home and prepare a nice dinner for my husband, my children, and me.

1999

I reached into my purse for my keys and felt a strange lumpy shape. I pulled it out and discovered a small brown cloth bag tied with a neat drawstring. Loosening the drawstring and upending the bag, several small stones tumbled out. Some were flat with rough edges, some polished round and smooth, some irregularly shaped with worn indentations. The variety of colors was striking: solid ebony, transparent white, mottled green, striated pink, clear blue.

Glenn was always surprising me with some unexpected token of his affection. He called them "shiny objects for his bride." I'd find a new book on my bedside table, a single rose on the vanity, a love note in my dresser drawer, a Calvin and Hobbes cartoon in the silverware caddy. But rocks? That was particularly strange. I handled each one a moment or two, enjoying their smooth, cool surfaces, and then dropped them one by one back into the bag.

I called Glenn. "Thanks for the unusual gift," I said. "They're beautiful."

"I know how you are about textures, so I thought these might help you relax," he said.

A year and a half had passed since I'd gone to Duke. When I left there, I'd resolved to return as their best success story ever. Crowds would part as I walked down the hall! Bands would play! People would point and shout, "Halleluiah!" I would be the perfect client, returning in victory and basking in admiration.

Well, it didn't happen.

The first twelve months had gone relatively well. I still struggled with intense cravings, but was determined to stay "present" and ride them out as much as possible. I averted some binges, but most of my success came from being able to cut binges short. Understanding the biology behind the binges was a huge help, as was the emotional growth I'd experienced. I no longer associated shame with eating, or even with bingeing. I definitely regretted any binge, but no longer attached a value judgment to the behavior. I saw the binges for what they were: biochemical blips on the radar. As a result, they didn't turn into the massive extended binge extravaganzas I'd experienced in the past, the ones I called *grand mal binges* that went on for months. Now, the ones I had were *petit-mal* versions that lasted for one sitting only or, at most, a few days.

My struggle was intense and never-ending, however. By the end of the first year, I'd become tired and discouraged, and felt myself slipping. Then, in the next six-months, I started bingeing more frequently. Though still able to shorten binges, I emerged from each one more and more irritable, angry, and frustrated. It seemed like I was beginning to move in reverse.

"I know what I have to do," I kept telling Glenn. "I have to find a way to stop the binges before they begin." It was no longer enough to reduce the time spent within each binge; I had to find a way to decrease their number.

I had learned how to try to avert a binge when a craving hit: go for a walk, take a shower, read, listen to music, deep breathe, do needlework, call a friend. The list of distracters was endless.

The only problem was, by the time I could *think* to do any of those things, I was already well into the binge. Only *after* alleviating anxiety with food could I think about what I needed to do to alleviate the anxiety I'd just alleviated with food! It was the old Catch-22 at work. When the cravings hit me, I was functioning in that damned amygdala where thought was by-passed.

The challenge was to get out of that primitive, non-thinking part of the brain, which is where the intensity of the craving resides, and into the thinking brain where solutions are possible. I'd been depending on my thinking brain to remind me to take a walk or call a friend or do any of the other options instead of eating. The heart of the problem, however, was that those options were essentially unavailable to me until I could pause and think. Once I'd begun to binge it was too late to do anything but try to stop the binge from accelerating.

This is where the rocks Glenn had given me proved a godsend.

At first, I started to "play" with the rocks absent-mindedly, while watching TV or waiting at a traffic light. But I soon discovered that they helped calm me as I was coming out of a binge. In fact, they were so effective, that I scattered them about: in my purse, in the drawer of my nightstand, in the glove compartment of the car, in my office desk drawer. When anxious, I'd retrieve a stone and gently rub it. Sometimes I'd reach for the rough edge of a flat rock, but usually a cool feel and a smooth texture was what I needed. Then one day, after a crisis in my practice, I had a breakthrough.

As I cleaned the adhesive from around the edges of a brand-new porcelain veneer, I saw it. A hairline fracture in the lower right corner. Porcelain veneers are thin esthetic coverings for front teeth. They are extremely strong once they're cemented into place, but quite fragile to handle before then. After applying slightly too much pressure, I'd apparently fractured the porcelain on this veneer as I'd pressed it into place. This happens to every dentist who does many veneers, but today's error was especially bad timing.

Normally, I would have rescheduled my patient to return the next week, remove the damaged veneer, take a new impression, and make a temporary veneer for the patient to wear for the two weeks it took the laboratory to fabricate a new one. Embarrassing? Yes. Time consuming? Yes. But all would turn out well. This situation was much more complicated though. It was late Thursday afternoon and Sara was getting married on Sunday.

I took a deep breath, pushed the button on the patient chair to upright it, and rolled my own chair around to face Sara directly.

"Sara," I began, "We have a problem with this last veneer." I told her the bad news. "This fracture would hold until you return from your honeymoon, but I'm afraid it will show in photographs, so we'll have to get another one made before the wedding."

Sara fought back tears. "Is that possible? The wedding's in *three* days."

I took both of her hands in mine and said, "Look at me Sara." I waited until she raised her eyes to meet mine. "You've been my patient since you were three. You *will* have a beautiful smile on your wedding day. I'll have to keep you here today another hour or so, and I'll see you sometime Saturday, at whatever time will work for you."

"I can't come Saturday 'til after four."

"That will be fine. I'll arrange everything," I said as I reached for the tissue box on the counter and handed it to her. "I'm so sorry for this. I know you have better things to do than come to the dentist during these last few days before your wedding."

I knew Sara trusted me. I was making a big promise, and I could feel the tension in my chest mounting.

"Why don't you take a little bathroom break while I call the lab?"

I walked into my office and called the dental lab technician I'd been using for years. "Jimmy, I have a big favor to ask..."

Thank goodness Sara was the last patient of the day that Thursday.

And thank goodness for Hannelore, one of my loyal assistants for more than two decades. She didn't hesitate to stay late that Thursday or to come in on Saturday afternoon. We got the veneer placed successfully, and Sara sent me a wedding picture weeks later with a note attached: "Thank you for my smile."

After Sara and Hannelore went home that Saturday afternoon, I locked the door behind them and went into my private office. The tension I'd felt since Thursday crashed in on me. I went into autopilot. Without so much as a fleeting thought, my amygdala opened the bottom left drawer of my desk and reached under the manila folder where I had, in the past, kept a stash of candy. There I would find relief in the form of M&Ms or Kit-Kats or Snickers. Instead, I was startled when my fingers touched a hard, cool, smooth object. Pulling it out, I found one of the stones Glenn had given me.

I rolled it around in my hand several times, occupied with its smooth texture, connecting to the feel of it, when I realized the tension in my chest and shoulders was loosening. And without food! For the first time in my memory, something other than food had soothed me through that first intense moment of a craving.

This was a huge breakthrough!

From that day on, I found ways to keep my "worry stones" not only near me, but accessible at all times. I took them out of the glove compartment and put them into the cup-holder in my car; I took them out of the drawer of my nightstand and laid them within easy reach; I took them from my desk drawer and placed them in a beautiful ceramic bowl my daughter had made. I even carried one or two in my white clinic jacket. As soon as I felt any tension rising, I would touch a stone. They soothed and somehow grounded me, bringing me back from the land of the amygdala.

Since it was their texture that seemed to do the trick, I tried small pieces of silk, corduroy, cut velvet, polished cotton. I discovered a whole world of soothing touch. I'd never worn bracelets before, but suddenly found them a way to soothe. I shared with my friends and family how textures helped me, and I began to receive gifts of various materials.

With this knowledge in mind, I searched for other skills that could help me through the moment of anxiety and the crisis of the craving. I developed the acronym, TICKET, which became my way out of the non-thinking amygdala and into the thinking brain. My ticket takes me from blind reaction to a place where I can think and problem-solve.

T-I-C-K-E-T

The first three letters stand for quick actions I can do in the first split second of stress, *without thinking.* It required much repetition over a long period of time, but these actions eventually became automatic. I practiced when I wasn't stressed, when I wasn't craving. I'm convinced that I wouldn't have experienced the breakthrough that Saturday in my office if I hadn't already practiced using those stones to relieve minor tension. These actions don't work every time, but they lessen the power of the craving often enough to be of great benefit.

T for **Touch**. I touch something, anything. Touch is a primal way to soothe, and what I need most in that first moment of craving is to be soothed. Touch also brings me back to a more conscious state where I can think. That Saturday, the stones in my desk drawer helped me to think without eating, as opposed to eating without thinking. For me, touching a stone, or some other soothing object, is the first step out of an intense craving. Over time, I've found that even gently stroking the back of my hand brings comfort. I experimented with various objects and found that just about any texture is soothing to me as long as it's instantly available.

I for **Inhale**. I simply get air into my lungs. Fortunately for many people, this is the first thing they do in times of stress. I, on the other hand, rarely "remember" to breathe when I'm at the height of anxiety. My breathing gets very shallow and erratic. I suspect people who carry tension in their chest, as I do, find it harder to breathe through a stress than those who carry it elsewhere, such as in their heads, stomach, or shoulders.

I can't do a proper deep-breathing routine at this point. I just try to get air deep into my lungs. With time, I go into a more practiced breathing exercise, but in that first moment, I simply inhale. Putting my hand on my chest and feeling it rise as I inhale and relax as I exhale seems to help. I frequently say the word *relax* to myself on the exhalation.

It's been said that *breath is the bridge* between the craving and thinking. By changing my breathing from shallow and quick to slow and deep, I can break out of that automatic fight-or-flight mode. Deep, slow breathing sends a signal to my body that the emergency is passing.[1]

C for **Change**. I change seats, change channels, change a ring to a different finger. I cross or uncross my legs, fold or unfold my arms. I push my hair behind my ears, turn the light on or off, turn up the music on the car radio. The list is endless. I find that this step does more than anything else to bring me all the way back to the present. With change, we confuse the brain and, in the face of confusion, the brain tries to think.[2] And to get back to a thinking state is exactly what I need to do.

These first three actions, **T-I-C (Touch-Inhale-Change)**, have become second nature for me whenever I feel anxious. I touch, breathe, and change something all within a few seconds, and often simultaneously. These actions have become almost totally involuntary, like a physical *tic*.

We don't know whether adults can actually change their biochemistry or develop new neural pathways or not. From personal experience, however, I know that I can short-circuit the time I spend in the amygdala by taking the above three actions. I practice them often, when stressed or not, and every time I feel an urge. I am not able to keep from eating *every* time I have a craving, but, over time, my success rate has risen dramatically.

I quickly follow-up the first three steps, T-I-C (Touch-Inhale-Change), with the next three steps in the acronym, **K-E-T (Know-Enter-Tolerate)**:

K for **Know.** I now know that the intense craving will only last a few minutes and that I will not die if I don't act on it. Once I can think, the first thing I do is remind myself of that fact. Most people, myself included before I learned better, don't believe that the actual physical craving, if left to run its course, will remain only a few minutes. I remember the first time someone suggested that I wait out an intense craving. I thought they were insane. I honestly believed that the craving would last until I ate something. To watch it go away on its own was an extremely difficult, but powerful, lesson. I still remind myself of the transient nature of a craving when I am *not* in the throes of one. That makes it easier to believe when the cravings hit. *This too shall pass.*

E for **Enter.** I enter what I call the Eye of the Binge Storm. There is calm in the eye of a hurricane. So, too, there is a place of calm in the eye of the binge storm. This is where I seek solace until the stormy crisis has passed. The goal is to calm down and let the craving subside without eating, but when I'm in an intense craving, I can't conceive of *not* eating, so I tell myself to calm down enough to actually taste the food I so desperately want. In other words, I give myself permission to eat, but only after the craving has passed. I just need to stay in that safe place without bingeing long enough to be mindful of what I'm eating.

This step took a great deal of practice. At first, I was often in the middle of a binge before I was able to enter the eye of the storm; from there, I could at least slow down the binge. With time and practice, however, I was able to recognize the signs of a coming storm, get to that safe place, and avert the binge altogether.

Once I'm in that calm center, I can start controlled deep breathing. As I slow down my breathing, my body is convinced that the danger is passing; my body can let go of the anxiety. I stay in that place, breathing deeply, as long as needed. Sometimes I pace, but I try to walk more and more slowly as I calm my breathing. I visualize myself looking out at the storm around me, and remember I am safe.

At first, I almost always ate something after I calmed down, but not nearly as much as I would have had I dived right into a binge without thinking. Perhaps I needed to be convinced that I really would allow myself to eat. Now, I rarely need food after I have recovered from the anxiety.

T for Tolerate. Take time in that place of calm and learn to tolerate the discomfort, at least to some degree. I know this advice sounds strange, maybe even cruel, but through bingeing I had become accustomed to anesthetizing every negative experience. I needed to learn to tolerate some discomfort or I would have gone on numbing myself forever. It's a balancing act to decide which stresses can be eliminated, which can be soothed, and which must simply be tolerated. *Learn to ride that wave*, Patricia advised. Learning to surf the waves of anxiety was a painful, but potent, lesson.

Even if I eat when I'm in the throes of the craving, I still proceed through these steps. This accomplishes two crucial goals. First, the sequence becomes more automatic so it becomes easier to access it over time. Second, it helps break my natural all-or-nothing tendency. It's very tempting to call myself a failure and *not* follow-through. It's easy to tell myself *Next time—I'll succeed next time*. I still struggle hard to stay out of that trap. I've begun to learn from my stumbles as well as my successes.

We all have stressful days. I remember many, but one in particular is fresh on my mind—a day when I would have binged had I not had my TICKET strategy to get me safely out of the moment of the craving:

It's maddening. I'm busy writing chapter three of this book and fail to save my afternoon's work. Suddenly my computer beeps and the screen goes blank for no apparent reason. Just before it crashes, it mocks me with: *You may lose any unsaved work*. I blink, but I'm sure it also said: *You stupid idiot*! And I say...well never mind what *I* say!

I can't bear to start over right now, so I go to the mailbox to check the mail. Bills, only bills. I dash past the sprinkler, accidentally left on from last evening. I turn it off and come back into the house through the garage, only to realize that I'd left a window open in the guest bedroom all night and the carpet is soaked where the sprinkler had gently sprinkled, for the past twelve hours, gallons of water into the house. I call the carpet company. They say we must immediately pull up the carpet and cut out the pad so the sub-floor won't get ruined. When it all dries out, they can come and lay the carpet again. I try to figure out how all of this can get done before my sister, Brenda, who has not yet been to my new house, gets here next week. Glenn and I rip up the edge of the carpet. I suddenly realize I'm late picking up my grandsons from school. I grab my keys and dash out the door, leaving Glenn to remove the carpet pad. I'm half-way there before I remember it's Friday, and I don't pick them up on Fridays.

It's too much. I'm in overload, ready for Krispy Kreme!

Apparently my brain's on automatic because I'm already cruising on Smokey Park Highway where the nearest Krispy Kreme is located. How did I get here? It's not my regular route, but I'm only a mile from warm, sweet relief. And it's a convenient drive-thru, too. Life is tough, but I'm about to feel a lot better.

Yes, I'm on automatic, but now I switch to *another* automatic system at my disposal. I call on my **T-I-C-K-E-T**.

Touch: With my left hand, I grab a certain spot on my steering wheel—a rough textured spot, a spot I've reached for often. Then, with my right hand, I frantically reach into the cup-holder and find a flat stone.

Inhale: I take a breath.

Change: I throw my purse in the back seat and flip the visor down.

Know: *Ok, Hilda, keep breathing. It's just a craving. It will go away in a minute.*

No, it won't. Not this time. This time if I don't eat, I'll die.

No, you won't.

Yes, I will.

Go to that center of the storm. Stay there long enough to gather your wits. Then you can have the damned doughnuts.

Just four more blocks. Thank God!

Enter: *Krispy Kreme will not be moving in the next few minutes. Pull over and calm down. You want to taste them, don't you? Remember how you used to eat them. Don't go there.*

I pull into a parking lot and take a full deep breath.

Tolerate: I look at the clock.

Five minutes. Just take five minutes.
I hate this. It feels so awful.
Inhale. Exhale. Relax
Inhale...Exhale...Relax
I feel calmer. I'm coming off that steep slope.
Inhale..... Exhale..... Relax
Inhale........ Exhale........ Relax
I feel better. I can think. I can reason. Do I still want the doughnuts? Well, yes I do, but my supper plans include fresh salmon and roasted vegetables. If I eat those doughnuts, I won't enjoy dinner.

I'd still like a doughnut. Maybe while I'm preparing dinner Glenn can run out and pick up two for us to have with a cup of tea later. If he's through ripping up that carpet!

On another day I might not even consider letting doughnuts into my house. Or, I might go on to Krispy Kreme and have a petit-mal binge, but that doesn't happen very often any more. The point is, I have options now. I can use my TICKET and ride through the moment of a craving.

When I first started using my TICKET to get through the immediate crisis of a craving and get back to my thinking brain, I had a problem with what that thinking brain said to me. My inner critic was strong and berated me at every turn. Negative self-talk led to negative emotions which led to new waves of stress and cravings. My lost form that first week at the center, for example, had led to escalating stress.

Once I learned how to leave the amygdala and enter my thinking brain, the next step was to learn how to handle that inner critic. I had to develop skills to break the cycle of negative self-talk and negative emotions because I couldn't spend all my time fighting cravings in the moment, berating myself. That was simply too exhausting.

Chapter Six

Harpies and Siren Songs: Talk Back

1973

When I received my letter of acceptance into dental school I was ecstatic, but once I was actually there, I began to question my decision. I was swamped with classes every weekday from eight to five, and half a day on Saturday, plus all the studying and lab work at night and on week-ends. By the second week, I realized I didn't have the luxury of staying with a subject until I fully mastered it. I had to prioritize. I had to decide what to master and what to skim. The perfectionist in me hated learning this way.

On the day Dr. Schusler's infamous freshman dental anatomy lab was to start, I was terrified. Dr. Schusler's class took my stress to a whole new level. After retiring as a dentist in the military, he'd taught at the dental school for more than twenty years. He was a fixture around the dental college, the epitome of "old" school. He believed that women didn't belong in dentistry except as assistants. Dr. Schusler's open hostility toward females dominated all my experiences that first year.

Mary Lynne and I were the only women in the freshman class of just over fifty dental students. I'd been grateful when Jena, an African-American upperclassman, approached me at lunch a few days into the term. After introducing herself, she got right to the point. "Dr. Schusler asked me to give you and Mary Lynne a message. He said to tell you that he didn't want you females coming into class distracting his serious male students."

I stared in disbelief.

"What?" I was furious at him. And at her for delivering such a message. I knew for a fact that Mary Lynne and I were in the top three incoming freshman because we'd both been considered for a scholarship open only to students with the three highest GPAs.

"Does he think we're here to seduce his male students?" I asked. "I'm not looking for another husband. If anybody is, there are easier hunting grounds than here!"

My mind flashed on that grueling undergraduate organic chemistry class and the hard-earned A I'd received. And on the hell I'd put myself through while waiting for my final grade to come in the mail. "We *deserve* to be here." I said.

"Hey," Jena said, raising her hands in front of her. "Don't shoot the messenger. Personally, I'm done with the bastard." Jena's words checked my indignation. I could only guess what gauntlets she'd had to run, being female *and* black.

"Seriously, Hilda," Jena continued, "Don't give Schusler an excuse. He's brutal enough in his best mood, but angered, he can—and will—flunk you right out of this school. You'll do ok on his lecture exams, because that has to be graded objectively, but watch your back in his dental anatomy lab. It's all subjective. I don't know that any female has ever done more than barely pass the lab portion of his class."

I'd already sampled his lectures, and the bitter aftertaste was still with me. In the very first lecture, after about an hour of intense lecturing on dental anatomy, he'd flashed a provocative nude up on the screen. "Ok, boys, rest your tired eyes on *that* anatomy for a minute." Bawdy laughter erupted.

I was appalled. Surely he couldn't get away with that. Not in 1973. This was not a frat house!

Steeling my resolve, I'd visited the Dean of Student Affairs at lunch. I nervously told him what had happened. He listened politely and told me that that particular slide was just a "tension-breaker" that Dr. Schusler always used on the first day of class, and that I should probably just let it pass. "No harm done, right?"

"I guess not," I replied sheepishly, leaving his office, angry at myself for bringing it up in the first place. *You idiot. What were you thinking? Did you think they would change the good-ole-boy system just for you?*

But the desire to talk back to Dr. Schusler and to the Dean boiled inside me.

Things got worse. The next day, Dr. Schusler waited patiently with his back to the class as we all filed in and found our seats. Turning slowly to face the class, he said, "I understand a certain young lady in our class was offended yesterday by my slide illustrating the female anatomy." His bushy white eyebrows lifted high in mock dismay. "I am so sorry if you felt neglected." His voice dripped sarcasm. Picking up the remote, he clicked the button to bring up the first new slide of the day, and added, "So, today we will give the male anatomy equal time."

He then flashed the photo of a completely nude male stripper onto the giant screen. This time, the laughter was nervous and scattered.

So, with those incidents in the forefront of my mind, I entered Dr. Schusler's lab. My knees were weak and shaking as I found my lab bench. Thank goodness, it was against the wall and not in the line of fire, near the aisle.

"Now listen up, you pansies!" Dr. Schusler's voice boomed. "This is the class that will separate the men from the boys." He swaggered around the room, up and down the aisles. My heart pounded as he approached my bench. I wanted to look away, but it felt too dangerous. Staring directly at me, he continued, "Any God-damned sissies can leave now." You could hear a pin drop. "I take no prisoners."

My face burned with humiliation and anger, but I tried to show neither.

Mary Lynne and I studied together that night. Over the semester, we worked together often, doing wax carvings for that class over and over, brutally critiquing each other's work until it was perfect. We gave Dr. Schusler little room for criticism.

The year progressed through studies: neuroanatomy, physiology, biochemistry, microanatomy, dental materials. Dentistry filled my days and nights. I couldn't get the formaldehyde smell of the cadaver out of my hands and hair, or the images of dissected jaws out of my waking mind. At night, I dreamed of the slopes and angles, hills and valleys, cusps and contacts of molars and bicuspids. At the end of the first year, I made the Dean's List, but it was the B that I got in Dr. Schusler's dental anatomy lab that was the sweetest.

Still, I didn't feel like a success. At the end of almost every course, I felt less and less adequate. There was never time to master anything before it was time to move on to something new. Other students seemed to be building confidence; mine slipped lower and lower. The little voice inside of me kept repeating: *You are such a fraud.*

I hated the first two years of dental school. I never had another professor like Dr. Schusler, but I continued to feel inadequate. In our third year, we began to regularly attend patients, and I was much happier. Yet, I was still plagued with the feeling that I was deceiving everyone. That I would be found out at any moment. My inner critic haunted me: *You're such an idiot...How could you forget the insertion of the sternocleidomastoid muscle...What a fool...Watch your step or you'll reveal how stupid you really are...You'll be exposed for the fraud you know yourself to be.*

I kept my eye on the ultimate goal: my DMD, Doctor of Dental Medicine. Perseverance and consistent focus had always been my strong points. Unfortunately, I usually paid a high price. In this case, tremendous stress and a weight gain of over 50 pounds. For the four long years of dental school, I kept my head down and my nose to the grindstone, regularly sedating myself with food.

The Sunday before graduation from dental school, I attended Honor's Convocation. We all marched in. The slight sway of my purple tassel against the board of my graduation cap matched the swish of the long gown against my hosiery. As we took our seats, I strained to find my family. Seated in the front row of the balcony was Glenn, and to either side of him were our kids, Tim and Karen. Their beaming smiles and bright wide eyes told me how proud they were.

I sat there half listening to the speeches, my mind elsewhere. With the brass ring in sight, my psyche did what it did best: it second-guessed the wisdom of my choice in coming to dental school. Even though I was graduating near the top of my class, would I actually be a good dentist? Or was I just an imposter? And what about my family? I was the first *mother* to ever be admitted to my dental school. Had it been worth the price paid by my kids? Both the children seemed to thrive through those years, but had I really been paying enough attention to them?

We never employed a sitter. Glenn taught in a Montessori School where he could work the same hours as our kids, and went to graduate school on the GI Bill at night after I got home. I was convinced that he was a better father than I was a mother. I was glad that Glenn's calm, self-assured personality influenced them during those years. Of all the roles I've had in my life, motherhood was one of the most rewarding, but it was also the most distressing. I almost always felt inadequate. It was yet another area of my life where I felt inferior and incompetent.

The sound of my name suddenly jolted me back to the present. Ernest, sitting in the seat next to mine, nudged me. "Congratulations, Hilda" he whispered. In a daze, I stood up and walked to the stage to receive the Anesthesiology Award for "the graduating student most concerned with pain control and patient comfort." It was true: I felt empathy for everyone. Everyone, that is, except myself.

As I stepped onto the platform, I heard a young boy's voice from the balcony. "That's my mom!" I looked up to see Tim's waving hand and smiling face, so full of joy and enthusiasm. He was proud of his mom.

That was the joy and unadulterated pleasure I wanted to capture in my life. I wanted to quit hearing myself say how awful I was. I wanted to quit finding the negative in every decision I made. I wanted to feel as proud of myself as my son felt for me at that moment.

2000

May I join you?" the middle-aged woman asked politely.

"Sure. I'd love the company." The dining room at Duke would fill up shortly, but for now, most tables sat empty. "I've seen you around, but we haven't met. I'm Hilda."

The woman set her tray down next to mine. "I'm Abigail." She tossed her navy windbreaker across the back of the dining chair, and dropped into her seat. "Whee, I'm exhausted! I just came from the gym." Her graying hair was cut short, feathered around her plump red face. Sweat dampened the fringed edges. "I came in last week. How about you?" she asked.

"This is my first week of *this* visit," I answered. "But I'm a returnee. This is my third time back."

"Third time?" She emptied a Sweet 'n Low packet into her iced tea, stirred it, and took a long sip. I knew she was trying to decide how to ask her next question. As a returnee, I recognized the hesitation. "Uh, have you, like, uh, had to start over each time, or what?"

"No, not really" I said. "Some people do come back after gaining some weight, and I've certainly had my set-backs, but none of us are ever really starting over. We still have all the skills we've learned. Most of us come back just to keep learning *new* strategies."

"Has the program help you lose weight?" she asked

"Yes, it's been very helpful. I first came in early '98, and I'm down over 80 pounds. I try to visit every few years for reinforcement."

"Eighty pounds!! Wow! I just know I won't be able to do that." Her eyes darkened and her smile slowly vanished. "I have no willpower," she said. I could see her wilting, spiraling down. "I've never been able to reach any goal I've ever set."

I tried to be encouraging. "You'll be surprised at how much you'll learn while you're here."

"I'm only here for a total of two weeks," she said. "And I don't think I'll be able to come back any time soon. So whatever I'm going to learn will have to be this week." She looked discouraged as she continued. "I know two weeks isn't enough time to get it all, but I have no choice. Like the class on the inner critic tomorrow. My counselor recommended I take it, but I can't. I have a medical appointment that conflicts."

I finished the last bite of my veggie burger and removed the lid from a red Jell-O container. Shaking the bowl, I watched the red mound jiggle. I remembered when Patricia had recommended that class on the inner critic to me, and how much it helped. I felt bad for this woman who would miss out on that key message. Maybe I could help.

"If you have time after dinner tonight, I'll be glad to run through the basics of the class with you," I offered.

"Would you? Yes, I'd like that." She brightened a little. "Anybody who's lost 80 pounds must know her stuff."

"Well, it's an ongoing struggle for all of us, but maybe I can be of some help. Learning to talk back to that nasty little voice in your head is important. Back dining room at 7:30? Will that work?"

"I'll be there. No one here needs to shut that voice up more than me."

"I guarantee you I was right up there with you when I first came, and I still work hard at keeping negative thoughts from overwhelming me," I said.

After lunch, I buttoned up my sweater before venturing out into the chilly afternoon air. I walked across the street to my room, and made notes on important points to cover with Abigail. Since I didn't know how much she already knew, it was hard to know where to begin.

We wound up meeting together for three nights that week and we covered a lot of material. Our discussions benefited me as much as they did her. Talking with her about my inner critic, about negative thoughts and how I responded to them helped me to understand my own pattern of behavior more fully.

I think of the beginning of a craving as a sweet siren's song. If the voice of the craving resembles the sound of a *siren*, the voice of my inner critic resembles the harsh, rasping sound of a *harpy*. Both voices have to be dealt with.

For me, two critical moments come early in the process of dealing with cravings. First, I must resist the siren song in the immediate crisis of the craving, and do whatever I need to do to start thinking again. That is where my TICKET helps. But, even after I manage to slip away from the amygdala and into the thinking brain, I am still not safe. In the second critical moment, after I've starting thinking again, I must be wary of my harping inner critic. In the past, that screaming voice often sent me reeling back to the fight-or-flight mode, triggering a binge episode. Learning how to stop that cycle of negative self-talk and negative emotion was critical to my success.

What are the origins of our internal condemning voice? Certainly dysfunctional families where children are told (in both words and actions) that they are worthless can be a big part of self-condemnation. Also, studies show that some people may be genetically predisposed to a negative outlook while others are prone to a positive one.[1] At least part of this self-condemnation, however, is brought on by weight stigma that is so pervasive in our culture.

> *The fifth-grade children fidgeted in their seats as the teacher handed out drawings of six children. The drawings depicted one child with no visible disability, one leaning on crutches, one sitting in a wheelchair, one with no left hand, one with a facial disfigurement, and one who was visibly obese.*
>
> *"Class, I want you to look at these drawings and, without talking or showing anyone else, circle the picture of the child that you would most like to have as your friend."*
>
> *Giggling at first, the children soon settled down and took their task seriously. They were then asked to identify the child they liked second best, third best, and so forth on down the list until all six rankings were obtained.*

The obese child was least wanted as a friend. In fact, that child was chosen last more often than all the others combined.[2]

This study, done in 2001, was a repeat of a classic study done in 1961 with the same results, except that the new study reflected an even stronger bias against the obese child than the original study.[3]

Another prominent study documented weight prejudice in pre-school children who judged even a silhouette of an obese child as an undesirable playmate. When asked *why* they did not want this child as a playmate, the words used by these young preschoolers to describe the obese child were chilling: *mean, ugly, lazy, stupid, selfish, liar, cheater*. On the other hand, when asked about the average weight child, he or she was judged to be *smart, healthy, attractive, kind, happy.*[4]

Even these very young children had acquired the attitude that fat people are bad and, as such, should be shunned. The National Education Association's Nationwide Study of Bullying found that weight was the most common cause of bullying in schools (ahead of all other causes including sexual orientation, race, disability, and religion).[5]

Weight stigma is found in every age group, and permeates all areas of our society. Obese employees, for example, are often viewed as lazy, lacking in self-discipline, and less competent than their normal-weight peers.[6] Even health professionals, arguably the most educated about weight, often see the obese patient as less desirable than the normal weight patient. In one study, for example, 24% of nurses said they found the obese patient repulsive.[7] In another study, conducted at the University of Pennsylvania School of Medicine in 2003, more than 50% of the 620 primary care physicians surveyed viewed obese patients as awkward, unattractive, ugly, noncompliant; one-third of them characterized these patients as weak-willed, sloppy, or lazy.[8]

The idea that obesity is the result of a character flaw can be traced, at least in major part, to our cultural and religious heritage. Traditional American values of individualism and self-determination promote the idea that people are totally responsible for their life situations, that people get what they deserve. For thousands of years we have been taught that self-control is a virtue and gluttony a sin. Puritanical teachings, specifically the Protestant work ethic in which control and self-discipline is emphasized, have a powerful influence on our culture. An obese person, especially the "gluttonous" bingeing obese person, is seen as someone who lacks these basic values.[9]

The common stereotype of the obese individual, then, is that they are self-indulgent, lazy, and unintelligent; that people who binge on huge amounts of food must lack the will-power, intelligence, or motivation to change.[10] We internalize this in our very young years, and it is reinforced throughout our lives.

This stereotype is simply not accurate. Most of the people I have met with binge eating issues are motivated individuals who perform well in other aspects of their lives and are often found at the top of their academic classes and professions. In fact, there is a correlation between binge eating and high personal standards. One study examined perfectionism and binge eating disorder, and found that the obese binge-eating group scored significantly higher on perfectionism relating to personal standards than the obese non-binge eating group.[11] The high standards that those who binge set for themselves may, in fact, directly contribute to the bingeing behavior. Doctors, lawyers, heads of corporations, and owners of very profitable businesses are but a few examples of people I have known who are successful, but who suffer from binge eating.

Even though the stereotype is inaccurate, it is still deeply imbedded into our culture and into the psyche of the obese binge eater.

But whether the harpy's voice is brought on by our childhood experiences, by a genetic predisposition to negativism, or by cultural bias, it still must be dealt with.

I had to learn to filter through all the senseless and destructive chatter in my head and come to recognize my own authentic voice. Once I got to the thinking brain, I had to confront that inner critic and learn how to talk back. Otherwise, I couldn't work any plan, no matter how good the plan. So I learned how to cut my inner critic down to size. I ignored my father's warning "Don't you talk back, girl!" I learned to talk back. And often.

Before I could talk back, though, I had to know who it was I was dealing with. I had to *identify* my inner critic. It soon became apparent to me that my inner critic had her own vocabulary, favorite words she used to put me down.

Hers was the voice inside me whose favorite adverb was *so,* as in "You are *so* stupid." Not the one syllable *so,* or even the two-syllable *so-o,* but the one that goes for at least three syllables. "You are *so-o-o* stupid."

The *so-o-o* can modify any adjective so long as that adjective is derogatory or humiliating. The *so-o-o* is often accompanied by the word *always,* which stretches the personal characteristic into infinity and beyond. "You are *always* so-o-o stupid."

I came to recognize some of her favorites when she spoke to me:

> *You're always* so-o-o *weak!*
> *That was* so-o-o *ridiculous!*
> *You'll always be so-o-o fat!*
> *You're* so-o-o *irresponsible!*
> *How could you say something* so-o-o *insensitive?*
> *You're always* so-o-o *lame—what a failure!*

When she's at her most adept, she switches to my first person voice, as in, "I'm *so-o-o* sick of always being *so-o-o* weak and fat!" That's the infamous double *so-o-o* with its double derogatory adjective.

My inner critic also has a favorite adjective. *Bad.* It can modify any role in my life and usually uses the first person pronoun, as in:

> *I'm such a bad mother.*
> *I'm such a bad friend.*
> *What a bad sister I am.*

Over time, it became easier for me to recognize that voice. I began to separate it from the other, more reasonable and measured, voice in my head. This idea of separation was important for me. The more I envisioned my inner critic as distinct from *me*, the more I could confront it. I decided to give her a name. Since my inner critic was so malicious, I called her *Malisha*. She always knew what hurt the most and went for the jugular. Once I could call her by name, it was far easier to argue with her, to talk back. I got critical. I got loud. I got mad. I was convinced that Malisha meant to harm me, so I protected myself.

Malisha always seemed to taunt me when I was alone in the car. At first, I would turn the radio on, sing loudly, do whatever I needed to do to drown her out when she tried to talk me into fast food. Over time, however, I was able to use reason and logic against her.

Now, when I hear that voice in my head say, "You are so-o-o stupid," I don't take it lying down anymore. I don't just try to drown her out. I talk back, and with an attitude. I tell her that I'm *not* stupid. In fact, I'm actually quite bright. Sometimes I do or say stupid things. After all, I'm not perfect. But that doesn't make me stupid. It makes me human. I remind her that she is stuck in one of those deep neural ruts, and that I won't be pulled in after her.

Malisha is a master at all-or-nothing thinking. She convinced me that I was either perfect or a complete failure. And not just a failure at that moment, but for all times and places. I remind her that sweeping statements that apply to all times (past, present, and future) is, in itself, not very bright.

This all-or-nothing thinking is only one of many distorted and destructive thinking patterns that locked me in a world of self-reproach and self-loathing. For example, instead of describing my error, I would attach a negative label to myself and exaggerate its scope and importance. The way I stopped destructive thinking patterns was to confront and understand them with my thinking brain. By naming my inner critic and talking back to her, I was able to tease out those irrational, sweeping statements and challenge them rationally.

Psychology refers to the approach of confronting our thoughts and understanding how they affect our feelings and behaviors as *cognitive behavioral therapy (CBT).* By exploring patterns of thinking that lead to self-destructive actions, we can modify those patterns which, in turn, improves our coping abilities.[12]

Cognitive behavioral therapy is the most frequently studied, and the most widely used, psychotherapy for binge eating disorder.[13] CBT (especially when coupled with a good exercise program) has been shown to reduce stress and significantly reduce binge eating episodes.[14] When I found I was having a hard time squelching my inner critic, I turned to Patricia, my therapist, to help me. Many other people I have met with binge eating disorder have also found that a good therapist is invaluable in their quest for solutions.

We also can help each other. One day I was in a support group and we were talking about this idea of how awful our inner critic can be. A lady made a point that has stuck with me ever since. She said that she is a really good knitter; that she makes complicated sweaters and other items. "I have confidence in my knitting abilities," she said. "When I make a mistake and discover it after hours of working, I don't berate myself and say that I'm a terrible person or even a terrible knitter. I simply unravel back to the error, find out what I did wrong, correct the mistake, and move on. It would never cross my mind to doubt my overall ability to knit or to say that I was a complete failure just because I dropped a stitch. Yet, no matter how much we've learned and no matter how far we've come, if we slip up and binge, we go all the way to 'I'm a complete failure.'"

Wow! Somehow her story let me see the absurdity of what I had let my inner critic do. I decided that I would start thinking of missteps on my program as simply "dropped stitches." I would "unravel back to the error, find out what I did wrong, correct the mistake, and move on."

Once I had named my inner critic and started talking back to her, however, I wasn't through with her. One day a wonderful thing happened. I made peace with her. This is how it first happened:

With each deep breath, my body melts deeper into the exercise mat on the floor of my bedroom. The back of my head, my shoulders, my hips, the heels of my feet, everything feels loose and relaxed. My routine for the last few years has been to exercise, stretch and relax to soothing music, then move into ten or fifteen minutes of quiet meditation.

I finish my new meditation tape and think to myself: *This is a good time to summon Malisha.*

I sit up and lean against the wall. I've begun initiating "conversations" with Malisha, admonishing her for being so hard on me. I decided not to give her the power to always begin communication between us. When I entered such debates in an upset state, I was on the defensive, and she had the advantage.

I close my eyes and think of Malisha. She hangs in the shadows, but I know she's always around.

Malisha, I begin. *You're so hateful and vindictive. I'm sick of your criticism every time I make a little mistake...*

Something's different today. Feeling so relaxed and at ease, I can't muster my usual ill feeling towards her. *Let's try a different tack,* I think. Instead of arguing and confronting her, I decide to just listen.

I use my kindest thoughts. *Malisha, why are you so hard on me? What have I done that is so bad that you have to humiliate and lash out at me so often?*

My eyes still closed, Malisha, who'd always kept her distance, seems to move in closer. I'm shocked to see that, in my mind's eye, she turns from the ugly adult harpy I'd always imagined her to be into a little girl of about seven or eight, with short dark wavy hair and dark lashes. She comes into focus.

Her face is full and healthy, with round pink cheeks. Her sad blue-green eyes look strangely familiar. I try to figure out where I've seen those eyes when, suddenly, tears well up in them and she begins to cry. Softly at first, then in a low mournful wail.

A small subterranean earthquake shifts my world. I suddenly understand that Malisha is, and always has been, a child. A sad, lonely, frightened child who's never felt loved and nurtured. She's a simple child who's been lashing out at me because I'm all she has, and she desperately needs my attention. She is *me*.

I hug her to me and I begin to cry as I rock back and forth, gently stroking the back of my hand.

It's ok, Malisha. Everything will be ok now.

I sat there for almost an hour, reassuring Malisha that I understood, and would always take care of her. Someone seeing me there, sitting alone, stroking my own hand and crying, rocking back and forth, might have thought me ready for an asylum. But that day was one of the most healing in my long journey back to health.

Dealing with Millie—that's what I call her now since I no longer see her as malicious, just young and willful—was a big part of how I discovered my own voice. Slowly, over time, I began to hear what that little girl was weeping for, what she needed from me and what I needed from her.

We have come to an agreement now: I am the adult who looks after her, and she's the child who entices me to play. I'm the rational thinking grown-up, living in a demanding, grown-up world; she's the innocent child who can play now. That child, safe at last, can have the childhood she was denied for more than fifty years. When I think about it, she's actually been very patient. I shouldn't be too hard on her; after all, she's only a child. I'm grateful she did me no more harm than talking ugly to me and encouraging me to eat doughnuts and ice cream.

She could just as easily have turned me into a cutter, or a drug addict, or a sexually promiscuous street child.

I'm better now at recognizing when she wants something from me. It may not be something that's good for either one of us (like a whole pizza or a half gallon of ice cream), but I can usually see what she really needs, which is most often love and comfort. Sometimes I take her to Baskin Robbins. I let her pick the flavor, but I choose the amount.

Rubbing the back of my hand has become a reassuring, soothing gesture that summons up an image of that little girl in me. I gently rub the area on the back of my hand near the thumb and index finger and am amazed at how calm I become.

I still have to scold Millie on occasion. Just recently, I had to speak sternly to her. She'd been bugging me all day to go to Panera's Bakery (our favorite). I had several errands to run, so I had to be in the car, where she acts out the most. I'm learning when to indulge in the simple pleasure of a treat and when to say *no*. That particular day was definitely a *no* day. I feared she would take me on a binge if I let her.

I'm not bargaining with you today.

She whined.

I stood firm. *I'm the adult and you're the child, and we are not going to Panera's. End of discussion.*

And it was.

I came to understand that neither the adult voice nor the child's voice in isolation served me well. As the child without its adult, I was out of control. As the adult without its child, I was all about responsibility. Before, when I could no longer bear the weight of that responsibility, I would let the child have full reign. And that usually meant a binge. I was turning into a hard, sad person whose only solace was escape through food. I was split right down the middle between responsibility and unleashed out-of-control behavior. It was only through uniting my adult and my child voices that I found my own authentic voice, and some balance in my life.

I practiced the skills that got me through the moment of the craving, the skills that silenced the sound of the siren. And I learned how to talk more productively to my inner critic, turning her from an enemy into an ally. Through it all, I also had to find solutions to the everyday challenges of eating and exercising and getting enough sleep, as well as enlisting the support of others and learning to relax and take it easy. Like Ariadne's golden cord, these new skills I was learning would be the golden threads that helped guide me from the labyrinth.

Chapter Seven

Five Golden Threads

1982

I reached out to Glenn as much to steady myself as to get his attention.

"What's wrong?" He turned to me, concern in his eyes.

My face hot, heart pounding, I could barely catch my breath. I sucked in air, and took a minute before I could respond. "I don't know. I walk a lot more than this at the office everyday."

We had just walked less than a city block from our home.

"We better go back," he said.

"Let's keep going. I'm ok."

"No," Glenn insisted. "You're not ok. You're as red as a beet and you can hardly breathe. We're going back *now*."

I relented, and we started back toward our house, but my breathing and heart rate worsened almost immediately. I began to cry. "I can't get back home."

Glenn steadied me as I sat down on the curb. My breathing improved a little. "I'll be right back with the car." He hurried off.

I couldn't stop the tears. I was only thirty-five. How could I not be able to walk a block?

Stress was not the issue. I was more relaxed than I'd been in years. Finishing dental school and starting my own practice had been liberating. My practice, now five years old, was thriving. The luxury of referring procedures I didn't care to do, such as root canals and oral surgery, was freeing. I was once again able to be a master at what I chose to do. Being the first female dentist to open her own practice in North Alabama had turned out to be a plus. I'd already become known as the "gentle lady dentist" who did excellent dentistry. The hours were long and hard, but I didn't mind. I sped along doing my work with a sense of accomplishment, feeling better about myself than I had in years. I had even lost some of the weight I'd gained in dental school. At work, I moved steadily from one treatment room to another, keeping up with the youngest of my staff. I thought I was in better shape than I'd been in for a while. I was wrong.

Just a few days earlier, Glenn and I had decided it was time to start some sort of exercise-for-health program. Practically every day the newspapers and TV had a new story on the benefits of exercise. The huge aerobic exercise movement that had started in the late '60s had reached its zenith. Bookstores were glutted with new books and tapes on aerobic fitness, aerobic dance, aerobic walking. We lived in a fitness-obsessed society, and Glenn and I could no longer ignore the fact that neither of us did any regular exercise. Walking seemed an easy beginning. I thought it would be a cinch to just walk for as long as I chose. After a few short weeks of walking, I would move on to a high intensity aerobics class. Right!

By the time Glenn returned with the car and we got back home, I'd recovered. The next day I called my physician for a complete physical. I needed answers.

In the doctor's waiting room, I thumbed through the out-dated magazines on the table beside me looking for anything recent, but found nothing but old entertainment news. I waited anxiously to see Dr. Petersen about the results of all the tests he'd ordered: blood work, EKG, and stress test.

When I gave up on finding any reading material, I strummed my fingers impatiently on my knees and turned my attention to a waiting room full of patients. The man three chairs down and across from me nervously twirled a pen and tapped his foot. *He needs a cigarette.* Two little blue-eyed, curly-headed blonde boys played with Lincoln Logs at a small table in the corner. The young mother seated near them kept looking up from *Parents Magazine* to check on her sons. She was young, beautiful, and thin. I shifted in the hard seat, crossed my legs, and turned my attention to an elderly lady across from me who clicked shiny needles around colorful yarn; her hands seemed to fly as she knitted. Never looking down, but staring straight ahead, she was apparently lost in some private worry.

A short, chubby, middle-aged nurse called my name, then led me into Dr. Petersen's private office. He motioned for me to sit across the desk from him.

"All your tests came back ok, Hilda," Dr. Petersen began. "Nothing organic is going on. No infection, no heart damage. In fact, your heart and lungs show no problems at all," he said.

"Then why did I give out before I walked even a block?"

"You're apparently running on very short spurts of energy at work and have poor endurance. I think you're functioning in an *an*aerobic mode most of the time rather than in an aerobic one."

"So what do I do about it?" I asked.

"You definitely need an exercise program, but the key for you is to start slowly."

"But how does that help me gain endurance?" I asked impatiently. "There's nothing wrong with my heart, so why not just push through?" I wanted to fix it and fix it now.

"Your goal should be to get your body to start using *oxygen* when you exercise. It's running on emergency fuel, mostly adrenaline, and that doesn't take you very far. Your body needs to start burning some of that excess fat."

"But how?" I asked, embarrassed now.

"Start wearing a heart rate monitor and keep your heart rate down. Don't let it go above 150 beats per minute. Use a treadmill so you can stop when you need to."

"Ok, I'll give it my best." I stood to go.

"And Hilda, you know what else I'm going to say." And I did know because it was the same advice I'd been getting from doctors my whole adult life. "Lose some weight. The nurse will give you a copy of a 1000-calorie diet. Let me see you back in about eight weeks."

I took his advice. At least part of it. I bought a treadmill and a heart-rate monitor and started exercising.

My *resting* heart rate was an appallingly high 101 beats per minute. What frightened me most, however, was how fast my heart rate jumped to almost 200 when I walked briskly for only two or three minutes. I began my exercise program by walking only two minutes at the slowest pace the treadmill would go. Once I could keep my heart rate below 150 for two minutes, I added a third, then a fourth. I celebrated the day when I was able to stay on the treadmill for ten minutes with a steady heart rate of less than 150. It took me almost three months, exercising almost every day, to get there.

I didn't return to see Dr. Petersen in eight weeks, however, because I was embarrassed that I hadn't lost any weight. I tried to stay on the 1000 calorie plan, but simply couldn't. My reward for trying was a series of binge episodes, during which I regained all the weight I'd dropped since dental school. Dr. Petersen meant well, but, like so many other doctors, he simply didn't understand the costs of such a highly restrictive diet. Nor did I at that time. And I certainly didn't know that such a calorie-restrictive diet could actually trigger binge eating.

Even though I was beginning to realize what a toll inactivity and excess weight were taking on my body, it would be years before I could tackle my eating difficulties in a serious way and stay, long-term, with a regular exercise program. I got my wake-up call, but I continued to hit the snooze button for many years to come.

2001

The light on the digital clock flashed at me in a rhythm close to that of my heart beat. The number moved from 4:05 to 4:06 am. I'd tossed and turned and tried to sleep for almost two hours after awakening from a nightmare. *Time to give up and get up*, I thought. I'd always been plagued with nightmares and bouts of insomnia that worsened when I ate poorly or stopped exercising. And I had done both in the last several weeks.

As I slid out from under the sheet and light-weight blanket, I tucked them, warm from my body, against Glenn's back. I tiptoed into the bathroom and quietly closed the door behind me. I stepped resolutely onto the scales. My weight, while no longer my primary focus, was a tangible barometer that alerted me when mindless bingeing slipped back into my routine. I was not really surprised at the 10 pounds I'd gained in just a few weeks.

It wasn't that I had a set weight goal in mind anymore, but the excess weight I still carried kept me from feeling as healthy and mobile as I wanted to feel. I'd moved fairly steadily from my high of over 300 pounds to just over 200, but had started vacillating 10 or 15 pounds up and down for almost a year. Both binge control and my up-and-down weight concerned me.

I was also tired of the nightmares that had worsened in the last year. Certain themes figured prominently in all of them: I was chased, beaten, and raped or one of my children was in grave danger and I was incapacitated. I had to stand by helplessly and watch as my children were brutalized. The nightmares had slowed down considerably since I'd started working with a therapist. But, in the last year, I'd had a long bout of especially devastating dreams. And with each round of nightmares came increased bingeing—and a weight gain.

I returned to bed, switched on a small reading light so as not to awaken Glenn, pulled my journal from the drawer in my bedside table, and flipped it open to see what I'd written last. The entry, dated just a few weeks earlier, described my last nightmare:

Last night's nightmare began as a sweet dream… I float gracefully across the stage in a filmy nightgown. An orchestra plays soft music. All my family and friends sit in the audience watching my performance.

They tell me to jump. At first I'm afraid, but their cheering grows louder and more insistent. They shout that they will catch me. As the orchestra's music turns into a pounding symphony, I find the courage to take flight. I jump. But, in mid-air, I watch with horror as the crowd's cheering turns to mocking laughter; their previously sweet faces become distorted.

Suddenly, the crowd parts, and they point in unison to what they all conspired to conceal. I'm jumping, then falling, into a fiery pit.

As I fall, I'm suddenly transported in my dream to a dark alley. I hear my infant daughter cry. I'm hysterical to find her. "I'm here, Karen. Where are you?"

From out of a dark doorway steps a huge man with a thick black beard and sharp rotted teeth, carrying my daughter under one arm with a knife menacingly close to her throat.

He laughs and tells me to come and get her, but when I reach out for her, I have no arms, only bloody nubs. "No! No!" I sob. "Give me my baby."

I'm helpless. I can't save my own child.

More than two months had passed since that nightmare, but I shiver. I'd awakened from the dream, sobbing and flailing my arms about. Glenn had tried to soothe me, "Shh. It was just another dream." But I couldn't be comforted then, and I found no comfort now as I remembered the dream.

I finished reading the entry:

Why am I having these nightmares again? I'm not stressed. In fact, I'm feeling really good about lots of things. I've sold the practice, have time for family. I rarely binge and am back down to 199. I finally broke that elusive 200-pound mark again.

Again?? Hmm...

I quickly flipped back to the entries of my previous three nightmares. In each instance, the nightmares came within a day or two of dropping just below 200 pounds. After the nightmares, I invariably gained a little weight and the nightmares stopped. What the heck was going on? Was 200 pounds simply a physical-based plateau and the nightmares were coincidental to it? Or was some sort of psychological barrier holding me back from a weight that felt better?

I remembered that each time I emerged from those dreams, I had the same thought. Not a thought really, but a flash. Much like the flicker of a firefly out of the corner of my eye, or a creak I hear when I'm half asleep. Just a quick impression, but when I look and listen, I suppose it wasn't there at all. That fleeting fragment of a thought was: *I must gain some weight back.*

What was the connection between the nightmares and the need to regain weight? I resolved to simply maintain above 200 while I tried to figure it out.

Obesity is a painful burden, and is, in fact, what drove me to seek help in the first place. It is the primary reason bingers show up at centers such as the one I'd attended. Granted, the biggest reward of overcoming my eating disorder was to finally get rid of the shame and guilt associated with food and bingeing so I could move beyond a pre-occupation with weight and embrace the joy of a more fulfilling life, but while I was on that journey, I clung to the hope of a permanent change in my extreme obesity. Slow, safe, even unsteady weight loss would do, but I needed hope that I could lose weight and keep it off. When I was younger, it was all about how I looked; now I feared for my health.

Many experts on binge eating feel strongly that binge eating issues *and* weight loss cannot—and should not—be addressed at the same time. I disagree. At first, I disagreed on principle: I simply *had* to believe I could lose weight. Now I disagree on personal and empirical evidence. I lost weight at the same time that I dealt with the problem of binge eating, and so have many other men and women. However, if I had to choose between dealing with weight or dealing with bingeing—and some people have to make that choice—then I would choose dealing with bingeing. It is far more important, and yielded me far more satisfaction and peace, than weight loss.

All those who binge must find the path that works best for them. I believe that many, perhaps most, people who binge can deal with the behavior of bingeing *and* weight loss simultaneously as long as the primary emphasis is always on the behavior and not the weight loss. Some may choose to tackle only the binge eating behavior before even thinking about their weight, and that is certainly a reasonable option.

I agree with those who say that we have placed way too much emphasis on weight. After all, recent studies show that the healthiest group of people (the group with the greatest longevity and the least health issues) are those in the overweight and grade one obesity categories. Those with a Body Mass Index of 25-35 are actually healthier and live longer than the "normal" weight BMI group.[1] However, extremes of weight (on both ends) matter. Those who are underweight and those who are severely obese have the highest mortality and the most health issues.[2]

I always like to point out that if an eighty-pound anorexic patient shows up for treatment, her medical needs are addressed (even with an IV and feeding tube if necessary). Dealing with her extreme under-weight is a valid part of her treatment. So why is the extreme *over-weight* of many BED patients not addressed with the same gravity? I think that in an effort to stop making weight the *primary* goal, the pendulum has swung too far in the opposite direction and somehow has made even talking about losing weight taboo in some quarters.

There is also a very practical reason to deal with obesity at the same time we work on binge behavior. A healthy weight loss program always involves better eating and appropriate exercise which in turn leads to better blood sugar, better sleep, and better mood regulation. All of these benefits have a huge impact on our ability to control bingeing. For me, dealing with both bingeing and weight at the same time had reciprocal benefits: (1) healthy eating and exercise in an effort to lose weight aided me in reducing binges and (2) reducing the number and severity of binge episodes helped me lose weight. But if I ever had a conflict between the two—as I did when I hit the nightmares/200-pound barrier—dealing with the bingeing issue always took precedent.

In addition to all the work I did to understand what was going on in my psyche, I also made practical lifetime changes in my daily routine. These changes in lifestyle were all aimed *primarily* at reducing the number and severity of binge episodes, but I also kept weight loss in mind. I was convinced that if I stayed focused on solving the binge problem and made some practical changes in my daily routine that weight loss would follow. And it did.

The most significant lifestyle changes I've made involve what I call my Five Golden Threads: **Exercising for life**, **Eating for health**, **Eight hours of sleep**, **Enlisting support**, and **Easy does it**. Like the cord of golden threads that Ariadne gave Theseus, these Five Golden Threads have guided me in my effort to find my way out of the labyrinth of binge eating.

GOLDEN THREAD #1: EXERCISING FOR LIFE

I'm not fond of sweating, but for me one of the most important changes I made in my daily routine was regular exercise. To be honest, I didn't have bingeing in mind when I first started exercising. I did it for the physical benefits which, in those early stages of my journey, meant one thing—losing weight. When I looked at the National Weight Control Registry (which is a forum that follows more than 10,000 people who have lost an average of more than 65 pounds and have kept it off for an average of five years or more), I found that the most common attribute among the registrants is regular exercise.[3] Given the dire statistics on weight loss and the tendency to regain what is lost, I found the Weight Control Registry a solid and inspiring source of information as I tried to get healthier.

I may have first turned to exercise for the weight loss, but it didn't take long for me to see that it had other, more far-reaching benefits as well. My overall mood improved and my anxiety and stress levels went down almost immediately which, in turn, helped reduce the frequency and severity of my binge episodes.

Studies support the observation that exercise significantly decreases binge episodes.[4] This makes perfect sense when you think about the fact that exercise releases powerful chemicals that reduce stress, and 80-90% of binges are immediately preceded by feelings of stress and anxiety.[5] There is also a high correlation between bingeing and depression.[6] Some studies show that exercise can be as effective as medication for the treatment of depression.[7]

Nothing I do, with the possible exception of mindfulness meditation, does more to control my bingeing than regular exercise. I believe, at least for me, that it is virtually impossible to remain binge-free without exercise.

My routine today is to do some form of aerobic exercise (usually walking or elliptical) for 30 to 45 minutes five days a week, strength training a few times a week, and stretching every time I exercise. But the real key for me is simply staying more active and trying to remain in touch with my body.

I will always remember the first vacation our family took that involved physical movement other than raising our forks to our mouths! I'd worked up to thirty minutes of exercise at a time when Glenn and I decided to take our extended family to a mountain lodge that offered rafting and a very challenging high ropes course. I was tired of putting off all the fun stuff until I lost weight. I still weighed almost 240 pounds at the time and was not exactly light on my feet, but I did it all. I shot the rapids and lived to tell about it! I even finished the high ropes course by jumping from a fifty-foot platform to grab a trapeze (I was attached to a safety harness, of course). It was both terrifying and exhilarating. I regained some much needed confidence in my own body on that family vacation.

As I continued to step out of my comfort zone over the next several years, I learned to trust my body more.

GOLDEN THREAD #2: EATING FOR HEALTH

Since this is the story of my struggle with binge *eating,* it may seem strange that I wait until this late to address the issue of food. But food was *not* the central problem in my binge eating. I binged to satisfy other unmet needs.

I remind myself often that restrictive dieting is the enemy when it comes to binge eating. When I stopped eating primarily for weight loss and started emphasizing health, I changed the pattern of my eating so I could reduce the risk of bingeing. I still wanted to lose weight, but I changed my goal from reaching an ideal weight to moving toward a healthier body.

My new eating pattern became flexible, adaptable and moderate—words not easily written by someone who binges.

The three most important areas of food consumption that I addressed—and continue to address—in order to reduce the number and severity of binge episodes are: (1) changing HOW I eat, (2) incorporating STRUCTURE into my eating, and (3) MONITORING what I eat.

First, and perhaps most important, I altered **how** I ate. In the past, especially in a binge, I'd eaten mindlessly, rapidly, alone, secretively, and with shame and guilt. Now I eat slowly and mindfully, frequently with others, and without shame or guilt. I choose beautiful, pleasant surroundings, often with soft music and good conversation. I pay attention to *all* the areas of food that give me satisfaction. Not just taste, but also the texture, the smell, the sight, the sound.

This mindful way of eating awakened my awareness of the pleasures of eating. For most of my life, I'd either wolfed down my food, paying absolutely no attention to what and how much I ate, OR I'd restricted every bite I took. I'd been eating this way for so long that I had completely lost touch with how much pleasure food can bring. Now I've discovered my appetite again and it feels great.

A second important change I made was to incorporate **structure** into my eating. Disordered, chaotic, unstructured food consumption is the hallmark of binge eating.[8] Even when I wasn't actively bingeing, my eating was often still chaotic. I would skip meals, eat at crazy hours, or sometimes consume only one type of food, like grapefruit or tuna, for weeks at a time.

Some people argue that it isn't necessary to have a plan of structured eating, saying it's more natural to simply eat what your body says it needs, eat it when you're hungry, and stop when you're full. I agree—in theory. However, eating by instinct (sometimes referred to as intuitive eating), is difficult in today's food-laden environment, and is especially complicated and problematic for chronic bingers like me. People who successfully overcome binge eating almost always do so by introducing structured eating into their lives—flexible, not rigid structure, but structure nonetheless.

Incorporating structured eating into my life meant I needed routine eating times. People who diet and binge over a long period of time often lose much of their natural ability to recognize hunger and fullness signals. The longer the history of dieting, the more difficult it is to regain those signals of hunger and satiety. For a long time, I recognized only two signals: famished and stuffed. When I reached the famished stage, it was too late to think logically, so I ate irrationally, to the point of being stuffed.

Since hunger is a common trigger for bingeing, I knew it was important not to let myself get overly hungry. But hunger cues were—and still are to a certain degree—a dilemma for me. With time and practice, I've been able to hone in on satiety cues, but the early stages of hunger are still hard for me to identify. The strategy that works best for me is to eat *before* I feel hungry and then concentrate on fullness and satisfaction, stopping short of being overly full.

Having structured times to eat also helps me psychologically: I know it won't be long before my next meal. When I binged, I ate all I possibly could in the shortest possible time period, knowing I would feel remorse later. This remorse would inevitably lead me to adopt new, more rigid, and more harmful rules. Rules like *I'll fast for three days,* or *I'll eat only a thousand calories a day until I lose 50 pounds,* or *I won't eat any sweets for a year.* Knowing that I would eat again in a few hours' time keeps me from having a condemned dieter's *last meal* mindset. It's easier not to eat the whole package when I can eat more from that package just a short time from now.

I experimented with different eating time schedules to see what kept me satisfied. I've found that a schedule of three meals and one or two snacks evenly spaced apart works well for me. Even when those meals and snacks are larger than they should be, I try to stick with routine eating times, starting with breakfast. Eating breakfast gets the blood sugar off to the right start and helps curb impulse snacking for the remainder of the day. Some people find five or six smaller meals throughout the day works for them, while others prefer three meals (and no snacks). I've decided there are no set rules that everyone should follow (except always eat breakfast). Some bodies simply require more frequent refueling than others.

In addition to routine eating times, structured eating also involves consuming a variety of foods. I eat from all the food groups, aiming to include several fruits and vegetables, some whole grains, good oils (like olive and canola), and at least a few servings of dairy and protein. I don't want to leave the impression that I am some sort of regimented health nut; some days I may eat nothing but pizza and be perfectly ok with that. It's just that my default eating is now wiser than it used to be.

This type of eating is not complicated. I spend very little time in the kitchen. Some of the sweetest words Glenn ever said to me were "Honey, you don't have to be a good cook." In our first year of marriage, I was trying to be everything at once and just couldn't "get" cooking. I still don't. I wish I loved to cook, just like I wish I loved to garden. But I don't like either. I watch my siblings with envy as they move gracefully about their kitchens, making scrumptious meals, experiencing something that is foreign to me.

I don't *have* to be a good cook, or even a fair cook, to make my world of eating work. I can broil or pan sear a piece of fish. I can steam or roast or stir-fry vegetables. I can make a salad. And I cook a mean pot of pinto beans. But mostly, I can boil water, open a can, or microwave a frozen dinner. I have discovered delicious frozen meals: Stouffer's, Amy's, and Michel Angelo are among my favorites, and all make delicious, healthy frozen meals. I also keep a good supply of canned and frozen vegetables and fruits on hand for when I don't want to cut up vegetables or even peel a peach. Yes, I am a very lazy cook. I never—and I do mean *never*—prepare a recipe that calls for more than one pot. That's my lifestyle and I don't plan to change that part of me, so I work with it.

I can't talk about what to eat without addressing so-called trigger foods. *Forbidden* or *trigger* foods presented a special challenge for me. A great deal of controversy exists about how to handle these foods. Some groups say that those of us who binge should avoid our trigger foods altogether, while others say we should have no forbidden foods. I say each of us should do what works best for us. For me, it is crucial that no food be altogether forbidden. I don't mean I go out and stock up on potato chips and Hostess Cakes to eat anytime the mood strikes. I have to *plan* for foods that have been a problem for me in the past and eat them in a controlled environment.

Ice cream, specifically Edy's French Silk ice cream, was one of my major binge foods. When I binged at home, I chose ice cream first. Understand, any food—even a bottle of ketchup— would do in a pinch, but if I could get it quickly enough, ice cream was my choice. It was nothing for me to eat an entire half-gallon at one sitting. In fact, I usually did. In the year prior to seeking help, I probably averaged eating close to a half-gallon of ice cream a day, every day.

To prevent feeling deprived, I needed to include ice cream in my eating plan. When I first started my program, I simply couldn't conceive of life without it. To include it safely, I decided to change as much about the way I ate it as possible.

I used to eat ice cream mindlessly, frequently right out of the carton, with the largest spoon I could find. I ate it quickly, rarely stopping until the whole carton was gone. I ate it alone and in secret, often in front of the television late at night after everyone had gone to bed. I associated great shame with many foods, but especially with ice cream. How could I change all that? How could I safely include ice cream in my food plan?

I knew I would be better off to keep it out of the house, and just go out for a scoop or two, but nothing satisfied like French Silk, and it was available only in grocery stores. So, my husband (by now you know he's my greatest supporter) provided me with a possible solution. We would keep French Silk ice cream in a freezer in the garage. I could request that he get me four ounces anytime I chose, although I tried to limit it to immediately after dinner.

I was nervous about trying this approach because, in the past, once I took the first bite, I couldn't stop. But it worked. Looking forward to that treat helped me eat better all day because I didn't feel deprived.

I ate my French Silk ice cream from a beautiful blue bowl Karen had made in a college ceramics class. I used a very small spoon. I ate it in Glenn's company, slowly, mindfully, with great pleasure, while listening to soothing music in the background. I ate it without guilt or remorse because it was simply part of my eating plan. Could I stop at four ounces? Mostly, yes. Did I ever eat more? Many times. If I felt I had to have more, then I simply asked Glenn to get it for me. He would do so without complaint, without judgment, without eye-rolling, without a look of are-*you-sure-you-should-have-more*? If I did get a second, a third, or more helpings, I continued to eat it mindfully, and refused to feel guilty.

That first year after I was diagnosed with binge eating disorder, I kept meticulous records on everything from food and exercise to my frame of mind. Over the first seven months, I averaged one serving of French Silk ice cream *six* days out of every week. Do I think having all that fat and sugar was good for me? No. But I'm convinced that having ice cream as part of my plan helped get me through those first critical months. By the way, even while eating ice cream almost every day, I still lost about five pounds a month in that first year. Most important of all, though, the number and severity of my binge episodes decreased dramatically.

Was I using that ice cream for emotional (as well as physical) satisfaction? Absolutely. My ultimate goal was to develop a wider range of mature coping skills and rely less on eating for comfort. By not excluding ice cream completely from my life, however, I was able to "use" it as a needed crutch while I worked on developing a more diverse set of coping skills.

I don't necessarily recommend that all bingers include their favorite binge foods in their eating plan. Perhaps there are safer ways to handle trigger foods, but this is what worked for me. I no longer crave ice cream on a regular basis. I still choose to have it occasionally, but now I usually go out for it. French Silk still tastes good to me, but I can take it or leave it.

I think there may be a difference in *psychological* and *physiological* trigger foods. They are probably highly interrelated: the foods our body physiologically need at certain times (such as carbohydrates in the female adolescent years) are probably the ones that got tied to emotional needs as well. This may be especially true if we tried to diet our way through those natural cravings during our teen years.

Early on, a binger can't be expected to know the difference between psychological and physiological trigger foods, but with time and healing many of us sort it out. Changes come at different stages of an individual's life. From talking with other recovering bingers, this aspect of our shared eating disorder seems to vary greatly from individual to individual.

In the beginning of my journey back to health, ice cream filled a huge psychological need. Today, I am more aware of physiological cravings. Now that I don't use the ice cream as an emotional comfort food (at least not often), I limit the combination of refined sugar and fat because they tend to set me up for increased, and more intense, cravings, sometimes lasting for weeks.

In addition to changing **how** I ate (mindfully, slowly, without shame) and incorporating **structure** (via routine eating times and adding variety including "forbidden foods"), I also had to consider **monitoring**.

I knew learning to eat with a different mindset as well as changing from chaotic to structured eating would both be hard. And it was. There was a lot to think about and a lot to change. However, the last area of eating for health— monitoring—should have been relatively easy for me. After all, I loved research, was a natural record-keeper, and had been keeping track of my food intake since my early teens. I had no idea how tough monitoring would really be when it was no longer a matter of dieting and counting calories!

Having a curious mindset, I wanted to know and understand what was happening in my body. Obviously, I kept track of when and how often I binged, but I wanted to know more than that. I wanted to know how much food I was taking in so I could look objectively at what my body needed and how it was using what I ate. Because I wanted to stop bingeing *and* move toward a healthier weight, I would need to deal with calories.

But how to do that without getting caught up into unhealthy dieting was the challenge. Certainly, for anyone to lose weight, more calories must be expended than consumed.

Since it is critical for those who tend to binge not to eat too little food (or binge episodes can result), eating somewhat fewer calories while not getting caught up in a diet mindset can be a tough line to walk. When I dieted, I had always kept my calories below a certain number (which varied depending on how desperate I was to lose weight), so I decided to do the opposite. Why not simply monitor what I ate, making sure my food intake stayed *above* a certain number of calories and then see what my body did?

But what should that bottom threshold be? Many "experts" will say a 1200-calorie-a-day diet is healthy. It may be healthy in the sense that 1200 calories can provide us with enough protein and the Recommended Daily Allowance of important nutrients, but that is as far as it goes. For the obese, it is an ineffective way to attempt to lose and maintain a steady weight, and has contributed to far more weight *gain* than weight *loss*. For those of us who struggle with binge eating, a 1200-calorie diet is a surefire way to fail every single time!

In one study of obese women, half the subjects were restricted to 1200 calories a day with some off-limit foods. The other half were encouraged to eat at least 1800 calories and were told they could eat all foods in moderation. At the end of one year, the 1800-calorie group had lost an average of three times more weight than the 1200-calorie group.[9] Researchers suspect that women in the lower calorie group probably felt deprived (due to a low calorie diet *and* the fact that some foods were off-limits) and were unable to stay on the diet, and when they went off program, they wound up eating far more than women in the higher calorie, less restricted group.

Many people, especially those who binge, think they can't lose weight if they don't severely limit calories, but rarely do they factor in the food consumed during binge episodes. After months of trying to eat a low calorie diet they are unable to prevent bingeing. They do not lose weight and erroneously conclude that they have to cut their food intake even more when, in actuality, they need to aim for a *higher* regular intake of food.

Since I had spent my life either starving or bingeing, I didn't know how much food was too little (and would trigger a binge) or how much was too much (and would lead to weight gain). So what I decided to do was to monitor what I ate, keeping track of calories and never let my calories go *below* 1600 at first and just see what would happen. I could then adjust accordingly. It made sense that as I was able to reduce my bingeing, I would take in fewer calories overall and would lose weight in the long run. I just needed to find the right balance for me.

Monitoring? No sweat. Simply writing down what I ate every day was no problem. No problem, that is, until I hit my first big binge about four months after returning from my month-long stay at Duke:

I wipe the sweat from my forehead with the back of my hand. My head throbs. The massive volume of food I just ate presses against my diaphragm. I can hardly breathe. I tug at my elastic waistband to give more room, but my stomach, miserably distended, remains rigid and unyielding. I feel queasy. My back aches. All I want to do is go to bed and sleep this off. Instead, I sit as upright as possible at my desk and continue to type... 12 glazed doughnuts, 8 Mrs. Field's chocolate chip cookies, 1/2 gallon of French Silk ice cream... I am humiliated, but still I type... 1/2 cup of Jif crunchy peanut butter, 1 bagel...

Yes, I had counted calories for almost as long as I could remember, but I'd always stopped counting when I got "off" a diet. I always waited until I went back on yet another restrictive program to begin recording again. This was the first time I'd ever written down out-of-control eating, and I didn't like it. I felt disgusted at seeing what I had just eaten.

Monitoring a binge is not easy. We don't want to face what we've eaten. Plus, sometimes, in our frenzy, we simply cannot remember what all we've had. But, after a binge, I record what I've eaten and how much, estimating when necessary. I set aside judgment, reminding myself that monitoring a binge is not about feeling guilty or trying to motivate through humiliation. In fact, just the opposite: it's about looking objectively at what we've eaten and putting it all into proper perspective.

Those of us who binge tend to have all-or-nothing personalities. We believe that a binge, such as the one I described above, will cause us to gain tons of weight. We immediately dive into the *I've-blown-it-so-I might-as-well-keep-going* monologue.

Monitoring made me look at reality. The total calorie count for that binge of ice cream, doughnuts, peanut butter, and cookies was about 10,000 calories. That is indeed a lot of calories to consume at one sitting but, since it takes 3,500 calories to gain a pound, those 10,000 calories meant I would gain about three pounds. If I had actually stepped on the scales soon after that binge, they might have shown a much greater gain because of water retention, not to mention the sheer volume of food in my gut. The actual fat gain, however, was about three pounds.

It is not one binge that makes and keeps us fat. It is the *continuation* of the binge cycle. Monitoring helps me by providing data that I can examine and look at objectively. When I binged that day in May, I'd already lost about 25 pounds. Three pounds was minimal compared to 25. I got right back on track and turned that binge into a minor misstep, "a dropped stitch." By understanding the actual weight gain caused by the binge instead of what my imagination had conjured up, my *I've-blown-it-so-I might-as-well-keep-going* all-or-nothing argument was diffused.

Monitoring also diminishes *just-one-bite-won't-hurt* thinking. Though I want to remain flexible, I remind myself that *just one* jelly doughnut only three times a week will result in a weight gain of over 12 pounds in a single year. Monitoring helps prevent both extremes. The huge binge never means as much weight gain as I initially expect and the *just-one* of anything invariably adds up to more calories than I anticipate. Monitoring keeps me following that middle ground between the two extremes of *I've-blown-it* and *just-one-bite.* I monitor what I eat in order to help control my distorted thinking that frequently leads me deeper into a binge.

Some experts recommend that those attempting to control bingeing forego keeping records of any kind because it might make them feel deprived and that might trigger bingeing. Some say it's especially important not to record the specifics of a binge, but rather to put that binge aside and simply start over. I agree that we need to move on, but only after we have recorded and objectively examined each incident as well as we can. It's not about *starting over*. It's about *continuing* on a path we've thoughtfully chosen.

Once I've monitored a binge and looked at it objectively, I check in with myself. *Why did I go there?* Maybe I'm able to decipher the reason and maybe I'm not, but if I listen closely to what's going on, I usually learn something important about myself. By recording my observations in a diary, over time I can usually discern a pattern. Anxiety about a family member leads me to crave ice cream; anger over an unfair bill or a rude driver means chips and dip; frustration over my writing makes doughnuts call my name.

The key to monitoring is to look objectively at what you eat and not let your food intake drop too low. Any type of monitoring will work. At first I kept track of my food with calories; now I frequently use the Weight Watcher point system. Some people count food groups. With time, some binge eaters are able to stop monitoring altogether. Now, after years of dealing with my binge problem, I have no need to strictly monitor when everything in my life is going smoothly. But let me get stressed and I need to go back to tracking my food.

GOLDEN THREAD #3: EIGHT HOURS OF SLEEP

When most people think about dealing with bingeing or about weight loss, they think of exercise and food consumption. They rarely think of sleep. But sleep plays a crucial role in both binge control and weight loss.

A few years ago, I experienced a major bout of insomnia, getting an average of only four or five hours of sleep a night for almost six months. Depression moved in, and I lost interest in most day-to-day activities that had engaged me in the past. I had retired by then, so I didn't have to worry about working, but I even stopped driving for fear of an accident. My cravings were unbelievably intense. Even after practicing all that I'd learned, I began bingeing often and had a massive relapse, gaining nearly 40 pounds, before I managed to find relief. Once I did begin sleeping again (with the short-term help of medication), I explored the literature on sleep and obesity, and found fascinating information.

Science has known for decades that a decrease in sleep can lead to glucose intolerance and to an increase in cortisol levels, which causes us to put on weight.[10] More recent research, however, takes the connection between sleep, obesity, and binge eating even further.

A study at Columbia University showed how the risk of obesity goes up dramatically as the number of hours of sleep goes down. Compared to people who get eight hours of sleep a night, those who get only six hours have a 23% increased risk for obesity; five hours of sleep takes the risk to 50%; those who get less than four hours of sleep have a 73% greater risk of obesity.[11]

Still other studies show *how* sleep deprivation influences obesity. Getting too little sleep disrupts two hormones. Study subjects who got less than five hours of sleep showed a decrease in the hormone leptin and an increase in the hormone ghrelin. Leptin signals us that we are full and should stop eating, so a decrease in leptin causes us to keep eating well past full. Ghrelin increases cravings. In this study, the sleep-deprived subjects craved calorie-dense, high fat/ high carbohydrates foods, and kept on eating them past normal satiety.[12]

So inadequate sleep works against us in two ways: we limit our ability to know that we are full *and* we crave more food, especially the most fattening kinds of food. Without enough good sleep, most people will binge to some degree. For those who are prone to bingeing, it is far more serious.

I don't take sleeplessness lightly. Good sleep supports my efforts to overcome binge eating, and poor sleep sabotages them. After looking at all these studies, my relapse during that bout with insomnia made perfect sense. I'd been looking for new psychological insights into why I had suddenly begun bingeing when all along it had a *physiological* cause.

No one thing is a panacea, but I now do everything I can to insure that I get enough good quality sleep: I'm on a sleep apnea machine; I sometimes use an early morning full-spectrum therapy light to help keep my sleep rhythm steady; I try to go to bed at the same time each night and get up at the same time each morning; I avoid foods that trigger poor sleep (for me that's preservatives or anything that even hints of caffeine); I keep my bedroom completely dark; I avoid depressing or negative TV close to bed-time; I practice deep breathing relaxation as soon as I get into bed. I value my sleep and protect it however I can.

GOLDEN THREAD #4: ENLISTING SUPPORT

I have always seen myself as a fiercely independent woman who got things done through her own hard work. When I was first diagnosed with binge eating disorder, I was sure I could take what I would learn and simply proceed to solve my problem on my own, by myself (or at least with only my husband as support). I was wrong. I was home from Duke only a few weeks when I realized, as the guy did in the movie *Jaws*, that I was going to need a bigger boat!

Once I realized the huge advantage to having other people and resources on my side, I enthusiastically embraced their help. In fact, the very act of accepting and appreciating what others could contribute was a positive step in my recovery. Now, I am humbled and grateful for the help of others.

Here are several support systems I have found useful over the last several years:

Primary personal support: Most people need at least one personal support person who will love and support them no matter where they are in their journey with binge eating (active bingeing, recovery, relapse, etc.). It should be someone who will unconditionally accept who you are and where you are. Even though they are concerned about you, they should be someone who can refrain from telling you *how* to fix your eating problem (unless you specifically ask them to do that). For me, this person is Glenn. But it need not be a spouse or significant other; it might be a sister, other family member, or a close friend. If you have absolutely no one you can turn to in your family or circle of friends, then a trusted therapist is all the more important. I have even met people who say their pet has been valuable as a source of unconditional acceptance.

Behavioral weight loss programs & eating disorder clinics: A behavioral weight loss program is the support where I got my jump-start. There are many facilities (either in-patient or outpatient) scattered throughout the country. If you choose to attend one, be sure its program is not just about weight loss. It must have a combination of medical, nutrition, exercise, and especially psychological components or it can actually do more harm than good.

This support is one of the most expensive that I mention here. Fortunately, financial help is becoming more and more available from insurance coverage now that binge eating disorder is recognized as an official eating disorder. I go through periods of feeling guilty about how much I've spent on the support I've needed over the last several years, but then I remind myself of how much money I've wasted on food. Plus, by now, my medical bills would probably have become astronomical due to illnesses I could have encountered due to my ever-failing health. I am, in fact, convinced that I would not be alive today if I had not found the help I needed.

Support groups: Weekly support from a group focused on health is important for me. Some cities have support groups specifically for binge eaters (usually headed by a therapist). Some people find a twelve-step program like Over-Eaters Anonymous (OA) to be beneficial. I personally find their principle that we must admit that we are powerless over food to be totally out of sync with my own beliefs, but many binge eaters have no problem with that.

Others, like myself, find Weight Watchers helpful. The Weight Watcher program is healthy and allows for great flexibility. If you use the points liberally (as I do), it is not a highly calorie-restrictive program. They also have a no-counting plan for those who prefer a more intuitive-eating approach. Weight Watchers is also very broad-based now, emphasizing behavior and personal growth as much as food intake. I attend meetings for the group support network and to help me stay aware of healthy eating and exercise.

Some people even form their own private support circle with other like-minded individuals. I say find whatever support group works for you.

Personal trainer, a gym, or in-home exercise equipment: When I first started getting in touch with my body, I used a personal trainer for a while since I knew next to nothing about how to exercise safely. I also had a treadmill at home so I could walk for short periods at a time. I now have an elliptical which I love. I sometimes go to an indoor pool. I use whatever resources I need to keep myself moving.

Journaling: I cannot emphasize enough the role personal journals have played in my own recovery. Reading my journals turned me into my own therapist at several points in my journey.

Psychotherapy: I was required to see a therapist when I went to Duke, and at first I went kicking and screaming to my appointments! By the time I had spent several sessions with the therapist, however, I was appalled at how little I knew about myself and about what my past had to do with binge eating. I feel I could not have made the journey back from binge eating without the therapy I received in those first few years.

There are many different psychotherapy treatments available for binge eating disorder: cognitive behavioral therapy, interpersonal therapy, dialectical behavioral therapy, guided self-help. Many of these show promise, but the one that has been studied and used the most with BED is cognitive behavioral therapy (CBT).[13] Of those who are treated with a course of CBT for binge eating disorder, between half and two-thirds either stop bingeing altogether or have significant reduction in their bingeing episodes.[14]

Dr. Cynthia Bulik, a well-known eating disorder expert, explains how CBT is used with BED patients:

> CBT uses well-documented techniques like self-monitoring (keeping track of your eating, your binge eating, your sleep, your moods, etc. in order to uncover patterns), thought and mood recognition (understanding what the thoughts and feelings are that trigger binges), cue recognition (identifying other triggers in the environment like conflict, stress, aggravation, and frustration), alternative reinforcers (finding other ways to soothe or reward yourself aside from food), chaining (unpacking what the sequence of events, thoughts, and feelings are that led up to the binge), thought restructuring (learning how to transform your thinking to support healthy behavior), and relapse prevention (how to keep it all from happening again).[15]

As I read this description recently, I was struck by how many of these techniques had unfolded in my own quest to overcome binge eating—and how helpful they had been. Techniques such as learning to self-soothe, unraveling my destructive thoughts and feelings, learning to deal with stress and conflict, and the habit of self-monitoring had all been invaluable in my journey back to health.

EMDR (which stands for Eye Movement Desensitization and Reprocessing) is another psychological treatment which proved helpful to me. As I began to uncover the depths of my disorder, I became aware that I had residual post-traumatic stress from early childhood experiences that resulted in really terrifying nightmares (as I described earlier). I researched and found that EMDR was being used with combat soldiers and rape victims and proved as beneficial as other psychotherapies in helping them overcome their post-traumatic stress disorder (PTSD).[16] EMDR is a fairly new, non-traditional therapy, but I tried it and it seemed to help. Granted it may not have been the EMDR because I was working on other things at the same time, but my nightmares stopped soon after I completed a course of EMDR therapy. The reason I mention this type of therapy is because so many people with binge eating disorder have a history of dysfunctional and traumatic childhoods. I know of no controlled study in which EMDR has been used with binge eating disorder, but it may be worth trying if you suffer as I did.

Medication: Since we know that BED is correlated to neurochemical issues in the brain, the idea that medications can help with binge eating is being explored. To date, only one drug, Vyvance (which is an amphetamine traditionally used for the treatment of ADHD), has been approved by the FDA for the treatment of BED. Drugs for other conditions that co-occur with BED (such as depression, anxiety, substance abuse, bi-polar) are also being studied and are, in fact, being used off-label by some physicians for the treatment of BED.

I have not used any of these drugs myself, but am fascinated by the idea that drugs which treat conditions that often accompany BED may have cross-over benefits. I have a personal interest in one particular medication because of a family member. I share his experience here as an example of how the field of BED medications are being explored at present.

My brother, Jim, has had issues with alcohol addiction his entire adult life. He abused alcohol for many years until he joined Alcoholics Anonymous (AA). He did as they suggested and took one day at a time, attending two, sometimes three, AA meetings a day in the beginning. His craving for alcohol, however, remained intense. He sought the help of a psychiatrist and tried several drugs to help him get through his misery. Through AA, he managed to stay sober for almost ten long years.

He describes those ten years as "the most miserable years of my life." He told me that he had to "white-knuckle it" through every day and didn't see how he could do that the rest of his life. Finally, his misery drove him back to alcohol.

For the next twenty years, he drank every day, this time avoiding hard liquor and using only beer. He consumed at least twelve beers a day in order to keep the intense cravings at bay. Through all those twenty years, though, he continued to wish he could be free of his addiction. Meanwhile, the habit was costly and it was also packing on the pounds.

In his search for possible solutions, Jim read about a drug called naltrexone which is being used to treat alcohol addiction. At the daily dosages usually prescribed, however, the list of side effects and toxicities over time concerned him. As he kept exploring, he came across a unique way it is being used in Europe called the Sinclair Method. In this method, the drug is not used every day, but rather a small dose is taken about an hour before drinking.

Naltrexone is an opioid-blocker. The theory is that, over time, the pleasure effect of alcohol is reduced in the reward centers of the brain; thus the desire to drink is quenched as the brain learns that alcohol no longer has the same effect.

Jim's physician prescribed the drug for him to use in the Sinclair manner. At first, there was no effect, but after about three months he noticed that he wasn't drinking every night and that he was drinking less at each sitting. Within a short span of time, it became weeks, then months, between drinking. His desire for alcohol was simply not there. Recently he decided to "test" the process by again taking naltrexone, then consuming alcohol. Amazingly, he had two beers and had no desire for more!

The effect of the drug may not hold and Jim's cravings for alcohol may return. But, for today, Jim is celebrating. "For the first time in my life, I am free of my alcohol addiction."

No one knows what the long-term effects will be or what side effects may pop up or which group of alcoholics it will benefit. For this reason, Jim has been reluctant to discuss his use of the drug with others in the family (we have three generations of alcoholics at present!) for fear that it might not have the same beneficial effect for them. He also fears that those who are presently abstinent might decide to try it and perhaps have irreparable damage done to their sobriety.

After he read a draft of my book, however, he discussed his use of the drug with me, speculating that it might benefit BED patients since my description of binge cravings sounded identical to his alcohol cravings. I had never heard of the drug, but his experience interested me because of the strong correlation between substance abuse and binge eating, and because the same part of the brain is involved in both.

Because my old nemesis, the amygdala, plays a critical role in binge eating behavior, it makes sense that opioid-blocking drugs may decrease binge eating by dampening our reactions there. Naltrexone has been studied in laboratory rats bred for bingeing, and the drug did, in fact, extinguish bingeing in those lab rats.[17]

Early studies indicate that naltrexone may decrease bingeing in humans, but they also show that it has fairly serious side effects when given at an effective daily dose. I heard one doctor at a recent seminar say he is prescribing naltrexone using the Sinclair Method with a very limited number of his BED patients. He finds that it is helping in about half of those taking it. What interested me was that he said the best results occur with patients who have a personal or strong family history of alcohol or other substance abuse.[18]

The potential use of medication for the treatment of binge eating disorder looks promising. I am eager to follow larger, more controlled clinical trials, with a special interest in opioid-blockers. This whole area of BED medications is in its infancy, however, and I would be very cautious about using any of these medications even with appropriate therapy and close supervision.

GOLDEN THREAD #5: EASY DOES IT

While the Golden Threads I have discussed so far—exercising for life, eating for health, eight hours of sleep, and enlisting support—are all important changes I made, none of them would have been possible without this last Golden Thread. It is the umbrella under which all the others became doable.

Like the majority of those who binge eat, my binge episodes most often come on the heels of stress, so I knew I would have to learn to deal with stress if I was going to decrease the frequency and severity of the binges. Learning to relax and take it easy was the single most important—and the most difficult—lifestyle change I made.

The idea that I could deal with my food issues without my teeth clenched and my fists raised was new to me. Adopting a more easy-going attitude required that I first learn to physically relax in the face of stressful situations. This skill was not easy and required time and practice to develop.

I knew that I had a hair-trigger stress response in my amygdala that sent me into a *fight-or-flight response* at the least provocation. I knew how our bodies gear up for action in the face of danger, either real or imagined: our chest tighten, our heart rate and blood pressure go up, our palms get sweaty, our breathing becomes rapid and shallow. I also understood that, once the perceived danger is gone, our body undergoes an *opposite* reaction called the *relaxation response*: our heart rate and blood pressure go down and our breathing returns to a deeper, slower pace. Stress dissipates.

What I had to learn and practice, however, was that the bridge between the fight-or-flight response and the relaxation response resides in the *breath*. When I could slow down my breathing and get more air in, the rest of the responses seemed to follow naturally: my heart rate slowed, the tightness in my chest lessened, the butterflies in my stomach dissipated. Just by purposely changing my breathing, I could cause my whole body and mind to relax.[19] That was an amazing realization and one that I use often.

Along with touching a soothing object, simply getting breath into my lungs usually gave immediate relief in the moment of stress. But sometimes, when I'm highly anxious, I have trouble accessing deep breathing. That's when I go back to basics. I place my hands on my chest or belly. As I inhale through my nose and take in more and more air, I concentrate on letting my chest and belly rise. The physical presence of my hands on my body makes me more aware of the action.

The top of the breath, when I have taken in air and have not yet begun to exhale, is where I begin to settle down. I stay there a few moments before releasing the air. Something very quiet and peaceful happens there, at that top of the breath. As I exhale slowly through pursed lips, I focus on letting my chest and belly fall inward. After a few cycles of this slow, practiced, deep breathing, I'm always calmer, always more relaxed, and always better able to handle whatever is coming at me.

I try to slip away from a tense situation—a stressful family encounter, an unproductive writing session, or an overloaded buffet table—to calm myself privately with this breathing technique. It can be done, of course, when others are around, but my preference is to be alone with my deep breathing whenever possible.

By practicing relaxation through deep breathing every day, I'm calmer and can *preclude* many of the distressful moments I used to face daily. This relaxation gives me a sense of quiet control, as opposed to the frantic feeling of being out-of-control, or even the oppressive feeling of forced control. Or maybe it is the sense that control is not needed at all.

Once I learned how to use controlled breathing to relax in the moment, I moved on to a skill that would not only help me overcome binge eating, but would prove life-changing. That skill was mindfulness.

For most of my life, I had been disengaged from myself and the world around me. Much of my disconnection could be traced back to my crazy childhood. In that early home, I was often forced to "disappear" both physically and emotionally in order to survive. An unconscious severance from myself had begun. I continued that disengagement into my adolescent years. Like so many young girls, I had shut down and disconnected from a body I loathed. I learned early to distance myself from a body that met no one's standards. Not society's standards of the perfect shape, not my own unrealistic standards of what it meant to be a beautiful woman.

Additionally, as a perfectionist, I often set impossibly high performance goals, and when I didn't meet them, I had to escape the inevitable sense of failure that followed. I kept running away from failure and from the person I'd become, a person I really didn't like. Everything worth having or being was somewhere out there in the future, waiting for me to lose weight, waiting for me to be acceptable, waiting for me to be perfect. Waiting. Always waiting. That attitude had denied me the pleasure of the moment.

All of these—my childhood, my body-hatred, my personality traits and attitudes—had resulted in a disconnection that bingeing facilitated. And, of course, the bingeing then cycled me into even deeper disconnection. It's no wonder I'd become a woman whose mind and spirit was so easily disengaged from her body. And from the *present.*

Sensory mindfulness was a skill I actively sought to develop. Once I decided I wanted to be *present,* even for the pain, I started learning how to be mindful of each moment.

As a part of a class on mindfulness, one of the instructors had recommended to the class that we try to isolate one sense, and experience it as totally as possible. I took her advice to heart. For fifteen minutes one day, I sat outside with my eyes closed. I paid total attention to only what I heard: the faint sound of a distant jet, car tires on asphalt, wind in the pines all around me, a child laughing somewhere in a neighborhood park, passing footsteps, the steady hum of the air conditioning unit behind me, the resonance of my own breathing. Really listening to all these sounds, sounds to which I normally paid no attention, made me feel more alive.

The next day, I did the same with sight, and the next, with smell.

The most interesting sensory experience, however, was the sense of touch. Again I sat outside and tried to notice only the *feel* of things. The heat from the sun warmed my hair, the fringe of my hair tickled my neck, the wool sweater I wore scratched my arms. I wiggled my toes inside my sneakers and realized my feet hurt. I dragged my fingers back and forth across the top of my thighs and realized I had a broken fingernail. I pressed my back against the patio chair and felt the cool metal slats through my clothes. Rubbing my left index finger over my thumbnail, I felt the minute ridges. Sliding my tongue slowly over my teeth, I could tell which ones were filled, which ones crowned, and which were natural.

I was like a newborn just awakening to the world around me. Through this experience, done over and over with the various senses, I became more conscious of my body, of *me*, as a presence in the world.

Most days now when I first wake up, I take a few minutes to orient myself in the world of my senses. I listen to the familiar sound of my husband's breathing and the whistle through his nose if he's still sleeping. I take in the lovely colors in the vase on my nightstand, or cringe at the pile of dirty laundry in the corner. But mostly, I remind myself that I live in a body. A body that is both separate from, yet connected to, the world in which I live. I pay attention to my head on the pillow, or an ache here and there. I listen to my own breathing, and remind myself that I'm alive. It's *my* skin, *my* brain, *my* muscles. And I should treat them kindly.

I even found a landmark study which concluded that patients with binge eating disorder who use mindfulness meditation have a significant decrease in their binge episodes.[20] Several earlier studies had shown that mindfulness and deep breathing relaxation techniques are valuable tools for dealing with anxiety and depression in general,[21] and with addictive behavior in particular,[22] but this study was the first to specifically address mindfulness and binge eating.

I've learned much in the last few years that reduced my escape through bingeing, but nothing has been more important than this new-found appreciation of myself and my ability to stay present and relaxed in the moment. This day-to-day relaxed reconnection with my body and with my surroundings was the center point around which all the other needed skills coalesced.

As I searched for positive ways to better care for myself, I realized that I rarely took time and energy just for me, or just for fun.

I've never been fond of frills. Pink ruffles and lavender lace have never appealed to me, and fancy jewelry and expensive make-up don't tempt me. Give me plain and simple, give me sensible, and I'm satisfied. As was my usual tendency, however, I'd gone too far. In the name of simplicity, I'd ignored *all* pampering, and as a result, I'd missed out on many of the physical pleasures and comforts that could have been available to me long ago. Learning to become aware of and loving the body I'm in was paramount for my emotional recovery. It was a big part of how I learned to take it easy.

I began to pamper myself and find comforts without resorting to food. M&M's is the ironic name I've given to some of my favorite ways of pampering. I've come to define them as delicious little treats that I deserve. Some pamper the body, some pamper the mind, and some the spirit. I engage in some of these treats regularly, others only rarely, but they all nourish me and help me take it easy. Here are a few:

Music: I have added lots of music to my life. I used to only tune in to easy listening and oldies, but now I'm open to bluegrass, country, classic, jazz. I exercise to music. I stretch to music. I take my own music to massages. I've even used music in surgery.

Memoirs and other books: I've loved to read since I first discovered the written word as a young child. When I went to dental school, however, I found I only had time for textbooks. Then there was reading to keep up with my profession. Retirement and taking up writing brought the pleasure of reading back to me. Getting lost in a good book pampers my spirit like nothing else can.

Massage: The concerned touch of a good massage therapist is one of the most nurturing things I do for myself. It is a powerful way to help me stay in touch with my body. Massage therapy can release pent-up emotions as our body connects to feelings. The first massage therapist I used on a regular basis was a recovering alcoholic, and he understood with his heart as well as his head how fragile I was sometimes. More than once, I cried through much of the session with him, and he treated me with gentleness and kindness. I will always be thankful for his gifted hands as I worked my way through those early years of recovery.

Manicures and pedicures: Once, when I was visiting my niece, Amy, she treated me to my first pedicure. I picked the brightest red I could find—I called it *slut red*—and I loved it! I could not believe how happy those toes made me. Every time I took a shower, or wore sandals, or slipped into socks, I smiled. I now get manicures and pedicures somewhat regularly. They don't seem nearly so frivolous as they once did.

Monopoly and other games: Monopoly has been my get-out-of-jail-free card on more than one occasion. Thank goodness my siblings and I had games growing up. Monopoly (and other games like blind-man's bluff, red light-green light, mother-may-I, jacks, and pick-up sticks) amounted to some sort of therapy in which we could express ourselves. When we played games, we were extremely competitive and loud, often aggressive; but we were also cooperative and empathetic, full of joy and laughter, and not a one of us ever cheated. We knew we could absolutely trust each other to be fair and honest.

Games may have taught me more about living than all the schooling I ever had. But with my busy lifestyle, I had neglected them. So when I started pampering myself more, which was just about the time my grandkids were coming along, I added back some of my favorites and shared them with my grandkids. I even took up coloring books. Now there are coloring books especially for adults and I have at least one in progress almost all the time.

Mud Pies: I add this little M&M because one day I made a comment about mud pies to some of my grandchildren, and they had no idea what I was talking about. Needless to say, we spent the afternoon elbow-deep in mud, rocks, pine cones, and berries. What a glorious afternoon!

Movies: In the middle of the afternoon, I sometimes like a good cry at the movies. Or a good laugh. Or the thrill of a mystery. Or a heart-stopping chase scene. I like just about any kind of movie now (except I still hate slashers). Glenn and I try to go to the movie theater at least every few weeks.

Making Love: Being overweight turns *us* off far more than it does our partners. The complaint that partners have of their overweight lover is not the weight, but that we tend to avoid sex because of self-consciousness. Once I learned to love my own body, I enjoyed sex far more than I did when I had a poor body image.

Solutions to binge eating behavior evolve slowly over a period of time for most of us. By learning to appreciate *me*, by having compassion and a loving attitude toward myself, I began to understand that binges do not diminish my value as a human being. They are not failures. I am not a failure. Riding the wave of a binge rather than being engulfed by it can be tricky at times. The secret lies in one's ability to relax and take it easy.

No learning curve or path to recovery forms a straight line. In fact, I've never met anyone in recovery from binge eating who followed a single straight line directly back to health. The labyrinth is convoluted and escape from it requires many twists and turns, including back-tracking. It takes time and patience to develop the wisdom to tease out what can be changed from what is not under our control. My Golden Threads are the lifestyle changes I developed around things that I can change. They have helped guide me out of the labyrinth of binge eating.

By the middle of 2001, I was healthier than I had been in years. My lipids were near normal, my resting heart rate had dropped from over 100 to the 70's, and my heart palpitations were gone. At 200 pounds, breathing and movement was so much easier for me than it had been at 300.

I hadn't destroyed my binge beast, but I had contained him. I'd learned to deal with intense cravings. I'd converted my inner critic into an inner ally, and by doing so had found my own voice. Exercise had become a part of my daily routine. No longer wasting time and energy with strict diets, I'd learned to eat for health. I learned to ask for help and put various support systems in place. I was becoming gentle and forgiving with myself and with others. These new skills and attitudes were the weapons I used to muzzle and bridle and tame the binge beast. I had him cornered and in shackles. With my new-found knowledge, I felt victorious. Strong and safe and protected by my shiny armor.

Real transformation, however, cannot occur through armor. Eventually I would be transformed in ways I could not even dream of. But first I had some important lessons to learn, lessons that I could learn only in the deepest, darkest recesses of the cave. Only after I stood stripped of my armor, utterly defenseless in the darkness of that cave, could I come to understand what lay beyond the taming of the beast.

PART IV

DANCING WITH MY SHADOW

Weary from his long battle, Theseus laid down to rest. His eyes grew heavy and the gentle veil of sleep descended upon him. After a long and restful sleep, the light of dawn awakened him, and he saw that the Minotaur had freed himself and retreated to the innermost bowels of the cave. The passage into that deep recess was dark and narrow, so narrow that no shrouded human could enter.

Theseus, determined to complete his mission, knew what he must do. Laying down his sword and removing his protective armor, he stripped himself of all possessions. Naked, unarmed, and defenseless, he crawled through the passage, slowly descending into the darkness to face the beast alone.

Chapter Eight

Lay Down the Armor: In Pursuit of Perfection

From an early age, perfectionism was a way of life for me. It was my protective shield against the world. It became one of my heaviest pieces of armor. By my late thirties, I was almost immobile from its weight.

> *This is my lot; for either still I find*
> *Some imperfection in the chosen theme,*
> *Or see of absolute accomplishment*
> *Much wanting, so much wanting, in myself,*
> *That I recoil and droop, and seek repose*
> *In listlessness from vain perplexity,*
> *Unprofitably traveling toward the grave,*
> *Like a false steward who hath much received*
> *And renders nothing back.*
>
> William Wordsworth
> *The Prelude, Book I*

1984

I squinted against the harsh sunlight as I stepped outside my dental office. I struggled into the green Volkswagen Bug I'd owned since before dental school, put my purse and sweater in the passenger seat beside me, and lay my head back to rest a moment. I'd felt exhausted for weeks, drained beyond anything I'd ever known.

My practice had outgrown its tiny space. Seven years of phenomenal growth had pushed the limits of the 750 square foot facility. Keeping up with the demanding workload had tested *my* limits as well. I'd extended office hours to accommodate the bulging patient base. In addition to seeing patients from eight to five, Monday through Friday, I now stayed until eight pm on Thursdays and worked half a day every Saturday. That was 48 hours of patient care, plus the time I put in on Saturday afternoons finishing up all my charts. The perfectionist in me would not let anything be held over until Monday. It was important that I start my week with everything in perfect order. It was getting harder and harder to do.

Work on my new office building would soon be completed. I was determined to hold everything together until I could get into the new 5000-square-foot facility with its eight treatment rooms. I had planned and designed it down to the last shelf and drawer. It would be perfect. My first associate would be joining me as soon as the building was complete.

With thoughts of the new building and all that it promised, I wearily turned the key in the ignition, and headed over to the new facility. I always became a bit schizophrenic when it came time to look at the new building, which I did almost every day. Part of me was exuberant; I loved the planning and the excitement of it all. Part of me, however, dreaded inspecting what had been done that day. I almost always found something wrong, something not done exactly according to specifications. I knew the contractor was sick of me, but he shouldn't have accepted the contract if he wasn't willing to follow the specs. I hated measuring every inch of new work every day, but I had to check to be sure it was being done right. The contractor, and even the architect who was being paid extra to oversee the project, didn't seem to think an inch here or there mattered. It did. I had written into the contract that I would not accept more than an inch off specs, and I was holding the architect, the contractor, and all subs to that standard.

The lowest bid on the building had been almost twice what the architect originally estimated, so our future was riding on my making this expansion work. Glenn and I were not chasing the American dream; we were running from poverty. We lived frugally compared to other dentists and saved far more than we spent, but it never felt like quite enough. Fear of losing our security was never far from our consciousness. Both our parents had lived through the Depression, and Glenn and I both could remember times of no electricity, no indoor plumbing, and little food. There was always the fear that we were only one bad month away from being destitute. And the cost of this new building, which was absolutely needed for my practice to continue to thrive, turned up the pressure considerably.

Over and over in the last few months, I kept reminding myself *I can do this. I can do anything for a short time.*

I arrived at the new building under construction, glad to see that all the workers had gone for the day. After examining the work that had been done in the last twenty-four hours, I closed my notebook, brushed the construction dust from my clothes, and once again got into my Bug. An oppressive wave of fatigue washed over me. I sat in my car, unable to muster the energy to drive home.

Red, yellow, and orange autumn leaves slowly drifted down in front of me. A slight breeze kept them afloat long after they should have reached the ground.

I envied those falling leaves. Oh, to slowly sink to the ground and rest. I was tired, bone tired. Tired of work, tired of having to keep up with everyone else's mistakes, tired of being tired. I loved life. Really, I did. But sometimes...

I knew I would never drive a few miles south and accidentally lose control of my car and drive off the Tennessee River Bridge. Would never take a handful of Percodan for which I could write my own prescription. Would never stay after work to turn off the safety valve and float away to a pleasant nitrous oxide-induced death. No, I would never do any of those things. I was way too responsible for that.

I needed to get home. I needed to start getting our house ready to put on the market. We had decided to build a new home on several acres we'd bought in Lacey's Spring a few years earlier. I wanted to spend time with Karen, now fifteen and in mourning after splitting with her boyfriend. Tim was now a senior in high school and there was the state basketball playoffs coming up, the last college tour to be planned, and the senior class trip to think about. His graduation wasn't that far off, which reminded me that I'd volunteered to head my own high school class's twentieth-year reunion to be held the next summer.

I turned the key in the ignition and headed to the nearest fast food. Relief for a weariness I couldn't escape was just a few blocks away, I felt better already. I could feel my energy rising in anticipation.

"Two Whoppers and two Cokes, please." I only wanted one Coke, but ordering a second drink was second nature to me by now. I mustn't let the stranger at the window suspect I was eating both Whoppers.

I unwrapped the first Whopper and wolfed down half of it before pulling out of the parking lot. I washed the rest down with half of a Coke. As I pulled into McDonald's across the Parkway, I threw my sweater over the remainder of the order so it wouldn't be seen when I ordered a Big Mac and fries. And another drink of course.

I then veered into Wal-Mart and parked away from the other cars. I finished the food, poured out what was left of the drinks, and discretely dropped the wrappings and empty drink containers beside the car. I frowned on people who littered, but I sometimes became one of them when I binged. I drove north on the Parkway even though we lived just a few blocks from Wal-Mart.

I bet Glenn and the kids would like some fresh warm doughnuts.

I ordered my usual two dozen: one dozen for the family and me, and another dozen just for me, to eat on the way home. As I left the drive-thru window, I opened one box and picked up the first warm, soft pastry. *Nothing soothes like Krispy Kreme.*

I was completely stuffed after eating eight, but I managed to finish off "my" dozen before approaching the last turn-off near home. No cars were in sight so I opened my window and threw the empty box into a ditch. Opening the second box, I took out two and placed them on the lid. Afraid my family would not believe that I could get home without eating at least a few, I always ate two from the second box.

The shadow of my hidden shame hung like an angry wound over my life; it had festered throughout the years as I learned more and more subtle ways of hiding my secret eating. The fear of anyone, even a stranger at the drive-thru, knowing my truth was unbearable. But the fear of being found out by my family was far greater. I carefully hid candy wrappers at the *bottom* of the garbage. I stuffed my purse with goodies and ate them in the bathroom after everyone had gone to bed. I hid food in my nightstand, dresser drawers, laundry room, anywhere safely out of sight.

I'd always made cakes for Tim and Karen's *real* birthdays, as opposed to the *imaginary* ones when I shopped at Peggy Ann's Bakery. I had a routine when I baked their cakes: I cut a two inch section out of the middle of each ten-inch cake and put the two halves together before frosting them. No one was ever the wiser because there sat a beautiful eight-inch cake. They didn't know I'd already eaten a ten-by-two inch strip of cake along with an extra batch of icing.

I was almost home. I looked at the two doughnuts and simply couldn't eat them. So I rolled down my window and threw them away, feeling the full weight of my shame.

Tomorrow. Tomorrow, I'll be perfect.

2001

What a mess! I stood in my living room, ankle-deep in water. The hose on our washing machine, which was located upstairs above the living room, had broken in the night, and we hadn't discovered the flood until morning. Everything was soaked—floors, ceilings, walls, furniture. Tens of thousands of dollars' worth of damage.

I grabbed the problem and set about solving it the way I'd always tackled problems in the past. My deeply ingrained perfectionism took over. Stay focused, stay in control of the situation, and it will be done right.

Looking back on those first few days after the incident, I pity the poor insurance agent, the repairmen, and any family member nearby. I might just as well have had a sign over my head that admonished those around me: *Put your hands in the air and step away from the lunatic!*

"Lighten up, Hilda. It's just walls and floors and furniture, not our lives," Glenn reminded me. But I turned away from his advice, sure that no one but me realized the scope of the mess, and of the clean-up that lay ahead. How would I ever get my house back in order?

I turned away, that is, until ten days into the repair when I found myself standing in front of the open refrigerator, scanning the shelves for something, anything, to put into my mouth. Glenn had gone to bed so I had the place all to myself, just the way I like it for a binge. The desire to eat was overwhelming, the urge rising with each passing moment. I reached for the carton of vanilla yogurt and the jar of blueberry jam. My amygdala was cued up and ready for action!

The touch of the cold carton, however, jarred me back to reality long enough to engage my thinking brain. I quickly shut the refrigerator door, hands shaking, heart racing, and went to the sink where I ran cold water over my hands and splashed my face. From there I went to the den and retrieved a stone which I rubbed for a few minutes, struggling to slow my breath and get air into my lungs. Then, after a long shower, I was calm. I returned to the den, practiced some deep breathing, and assessed the situation.

As I considered what triggered my urge to binge, I realized it wasn't the stress of the flood that had pushed me over the edge; it was my own unrelenting drive to get it all done to perfection. Visions of the unyielding efforts I'd expended years earlier when building my new dental office came vividly into focus. I didn't like what I saw. Why did everything have to be perfect—every nail, every tile, every section of dry-wall? Why did *I* have to be in perfect control of it all? Why could I not just trust the workers to take care of things I really knew nothing about? I realized I was sick of the word *perfect*!

I remembered yet another time and another *perfect*. It was 1954 and I was in the second grade:

I looked in the mirror, tucked in my neat white blouse, and straightened the waist band of my green plaid skirt. Skirt. S-K-I-R-T. Skirt. My bright yellow barrette with its hot pink flowers stood out against my dark hair. I was ready. Everything was perfect. Perfect. P-E-R-F-E-C-T. Perfect.

Spelling bees were uncommon at my old school, so I was glad Mrs. Orr, my 2nd grade teacher, had one every Friday. She said the practice would make us good spellers, but mostly I think she did it so our class would win the school's 2nd grade spelling bee.

I was always the last speller left standing on Fridays. On this day, all four of the 2nd grade classes competed in a spelling bee, and I was pretty sure I could win it for Mrs. Orr. The winner would get to compete in a school-wide spelling bee. This was a big deal at Webb Grammar School.

And so the 2nd grade spelling bee began. We all stood in a straight line as Mrs. Jones, one of the other 2nd grade teachers, called out the words. Round and round the spelling went, and one by one my fellow classmates missed words and had to sit down. Finally, Mary Jane and I were the only two left standing. After five more rounds, Mary Jane missed her word. I spelled it correctly. In order to be the winner, however, I had to correctly spell one more word.

I held my breath as Mrs. Jones called out, "world."

"World. W-O-R-L-D. World."

I'd done it! I was the winner! I would represent the whole 2nd grade in the big spelling bee. Mom and Dad would be so proud. I smiled from ear to ear.

"Time for recess now," Mrs. Jones announced. We all started out.

"Hilda," Mrs. Orr called to me. "How would you like to stay in with me today? We could practice for next Friday's big bee." She smiled and added, "I have a moon pie we could share."

"Yes, ma'am. I would like that."

She broke the moon pie and handed me half. I sat there, just me and my teacher, sharing her snack. At that moment, I must have been the happiest kid in the whole world. Everything was perfect. I had been perfect, and I was being rewarded for it.

She called out words and I spelled them. After a few dozen, she turned past several pages.

"Let's try some of the 4th grade words. Just for practice."

I continued to spell them correctly.

"Hilda, you're very smart. I'm eager to see how well you do against the older kids next week."

I could tell she was impressed, and I beamed. She looked up mischievously as she flipped all the way back to near the end of the book.

"Conquer," she said. "Bet you can't spell conquer."

And she was right. I responded slowly, "Conquer. C-O-N-Q-U--O--R?"

"Close. But no, it's E R. C-O-N-Q-U-E-R."

Not perfect. I was devastated. I had failed Mrs. Orr. To my great relief, twenty-five laughing, sweaty children bolted in. Recess was over. I took my seat and fought back tears for the rest of the afternoon.

Finally, the bell rang, and I could escape.

All the way home the tears flowed. Conquer. C-O-N-Q-U-E-R. C-O-N-Q-U-E-R. C-O-N-Q-U-E-R. *I kept spelling it over and over in my head. I should know that word. My heart was broken.* Now Mrs. Orr doesn't think I'm smart anymore.

When I got home, Mom asked me why I was crying. I told her I'd fallen and hurt my knee. I didn't tell her that I won the spelling bee. I didn't tell her that I couldn't spell conquer. *I didn't want her to know how dumb I was.*

I dreaded the next Friday. I couldn't bear the thought that everyone would see how stupid I was. But I shouldn't have worried. On Friday I woke up vomiting, with a terrible stomach ache, so I had to stay home.

And what made it all the worse was that the absence spoiled my perfect attendance record for the year.

Looking back, the stomach ache that had kept me home was clearly psychosomatic, but I didn't know it at the time—and I definitely would not have been able to spell *psychosomatic*.

In the week that followed my near-binge over the repairs for the water damage, I thought a lot about that spelling bee and the agony I'd felt because of it. I did a lot of deep breathing, handled quite a few stones, and took several hot showers. This wasn't the first time perfectionism had stolen pleasure in my life, but it was the first time I'd understood that bingeing was a direct result of it. I knew I'd have to give up *perfect* if I wanted to give up binge eating.

Slowly, over the course of the week, I changed my goals and turned the situation around. What had been an overwhelming task to be tackled perfectly became a pleasant opportunity to redecorate my home. And this time around, I took time to enjoy it. I found that with the release of *perfect* came an ability to trust others to do their job. I didn't return to the refrigerator in search of binge food for the remainder of the repair.

It's healthy to set high goals and to do one's best to achieve those goals. The human race as a whole, as well as the individual, benefits from the basic desire to always aim higher and higher. To reach toward perfection, to attempt to connect to the divine, may indeed be what separates us from other animals; it is part of what makes us human. This desire has kept humanity moving forward, sustaining the human race for thousands of years. Robert Browning said it best, "Ah, but a man's reach should exceed his grasp, or what's a heaven for?"[1]

A perfectionist is someone who strives to do just that, to reach beyond his grasp. If that were all, I'd be happy to call myself a perfectionist. Unfortunately, I often confused the goal of *aiming* for perfection with the act of actually *achieving* it. Perfection is rarely, if ever, actually achievable. My best was simply never good enough. No matter how monumental my effort, if the task was not done, and done perfectly, the effort itself counted for nothing. All-or-nothing. The trap that cheats us of the joy of life.

I was rarely satisfied with my accomplishments. Because I set unreasonably high goals, I frequently failed to achieve them. Even when I did meet my own high expectations, I always had a gnawing sense that the reason I'd succeeded was because I hadn't aimed high enough.

I looked at what I had *not* accomplished rather than at what I'd done well. A 99% on a test meant I'd missed something I should have known. Instead of taking pride in my 3.92 GPA in college, I was reminded of the six classes in which I'd gotten B's: world literature, cultural anthropology, English history, French, general chemistry, and bowling. No one, more than thirty years later, should be able to remember how many B's they got in college, much less be able to name the classes.

Setting unreasonably high goals and almost always failing in my own eyes, bred guilt which led to poor self-esteem. I would then set even higher goals to make myself feel more worthy. And so the cycle continued. Without academic and vocational success, I was nothing, undeserving of admiration, or even love. I kept on pushing for greater and greater accomplishments in order to feel worthy.

Many people who binge eat are highly competitive perfectionists whose mistakes gravely distress them.[2] The psychologist, Albert Bandura, explains that people who combine limited competencies, exacting standards, and socially unacceptable traits are often plagued with feelings of worthlessness.[3] Obese binge eaters meet this profile all too well: we keep "failing"/being incompetent at dieting, leading to a sense of inadequacy; we set exacting standards of self-evaluation; we are frowned on by society as socially "unacceptable" because of our weight.[4] Is it any wonder that we harbor a pervasive sense of worthlessness?

Perfectionists often have a hard time discriminating. We think every single task requires our all. Again, that all-or-nothing thinking. In certain arenas it is desirable to aim for perfection, as unattainable as that may be. In my dental practice, for example, I think all my patients wanted me to be a perfectionist when I filled or crowned a tooth. And how much more so in the case of a brain surgeon. Or a parachute manufacturer, for that matter.

Once I came to understand just how much perfectionism was exacting from my life, I decided to aim for *average* in some areas. I'm experiencing many new adventures now: I did a physically and mentally challenging ropes course, I've taken up bridge, and I'm writing this book. I would never have attempted any of these things before. I would have feared not doing any of them perfectly, of being the dreaded *average*. What a wonderfully freeing feeling: to know that sometimes average is good enough. I don't ever again want to miss the joy of participating in the big spelling bee because I'm afraid of missing a word.

Perfectionism may drive us to great achievement, but it also diminishes much of the joy in that achievement. Witness my spelling bee: what should have been a wonderful celebration of success turned out to be torment. And I almost missed the pleasure of redecorating my home.

I've changed the image of my path in life. I used to feel I was walking on a narrow ridge. One mishap and I would plunge into the ravine below. I was constantly falling and having to pull myself up the steep slope to start all over again. I wasted a great deal of energy trying to stay on the ridge, or struggling to get out of the ravine. Then I made a paradigm shift by visualizing the road I was on as a broad path in a slightly rising meadow. As long as I'm heading in the right direction, staying on or near the path, I don't need to be so exacting.

The technique of *successive approximation* in which I accept small steps and incremental improvement is the opposite of all-or-nothing goal setting and is now working for me. Each month, as I see an improvement in my exercise, if I can work out just five minutes longer, I move closer to better health. Each time I shorten a binge or lengthen the time between episodes, I approach my goal. Each time I celebrate *average*, I am triumphant.

I gave up will-power. In fact, I gave up my whole way of looking at challenges in life. It seemed that everything I'd ever accomplished resulted from a hard, exhausting, shoulder-to-the-grindstone, I'll-never-give-up kind of pushing. Grit my teeth, hold my breath, and keep trudging forward had been my way. I constantly told myself *I will do this*. Coming from my background, that can-do, pull-yourself-up-by-the-bootstraps mentality is often what allowed me to succeed. But at what price?

In my fifties, it dawned on me that what I got as a reward for this kind of thinking was not worth what I was paying. Most importantly, my unrelenting and unforgiving way of doing things was counterproductive. It did not alleviate the biggest pain in my life: the shame of binge eating. The more I *pushed* at dieting, and the more sheer will-power I tried to exert, the more I binged and the bigger I got.

I had to learn to be kind to myself, to be gentle, and forgiving. To allow myself to be imperfect. To finally exhale.

Now instead of *I must*, I say *I choose*.

For some people—heavy procrastinators or those afraid of a challenge—a certain amount of extra resolve and striving for perfection may be the answer. But not for me. What I needed was to let go of *perfect*.

Perfectionism was one of the heaviest burdens I carried that kept me locked in binge eating. But *perfect* was simply the offspring of something far more deadly, something about myself and my attitude that I would still have to confront in the most painful experience of my life. I discovered I had only laid down part of my armor.

Chapter Nine

Nobility in the Struggle: Accepting Vulnerability

1988

I stood, right hand above my head, right breast clamped between the cold glass sheets of the mammogram machine. This was the third view the radiologist had ordered, and I knew that couldn't be good.

When I was about ten, I'd gone through my Aunt Willie's dresser and found her breast prosthesis. The image of that fake breast and my aunt's lopsided chest now loomed in my mind. My apprehension was not eased by the young technician. Earlier cheerful and friendly, she was now matter-of-fact and business-like. *Does she know something I don't?*

"Ok, you can breathe again now, Dr. Lee," she said from behind her glass partition.

Breathe again? I thought as she released my breast from the vise. *Not likely. Not until I hear my mammogram is clear.*

I couldn't have breast cancer, not at forty-one! My Aunt Willie was the only relative I knew who'd had it. I struggled to push the image of her rubber prosthesis from my mind. All that would replace it, however, were images of the medical photographs from pathology class in dental school. Photographs of women with blanked out faces and no breasts, jagged scars in their place.

I re-dressed and sat down on the colorful cotton chintz sofa in the small private waiting room. After an eternity, Dr. Ray stuck his head in. I wished it were Jim or Paul or any of the other radiologists that I knew personally. "Hilda," said Dr. Ray, "come back to my office for a minute."

I followed him back to a small area where several mammograms were clipped to a series of large view boxes. "Have a seat," he said. "I pass by your dental building every day on my way to work. You have a beautiful facility. And Paul tells me you're a great dentist."

Oh, good. He knows I'm in medicine, and he's going to talk with me today and not make me wait for a call from my gynecologist.

As he shut the door behind us and took a seat beside me, his expression turned serious. I understood immediately the import of his solemn demeanor. I straightened my spine and steeled myself.

"I want to show you your film," he began...

As I struggled to emerge from the grog of anesthesia, I became aware of Glenn tenderly stroking my right hand, and Nancy holding my left. Nancy, who had been my friend and patient for years, was my surgeon today. My brain tried to focus on where I was and why I was so cold. As my thoughts aligned, I remembered that I was having a biopsy to test the mass Dr. Ray had found on my mammogram four days earlier. I'd made Nancy promise to talk to me as soon as I woke up. I couldn't bear the thought of waiting one second longer than necessary.

"I'm sorry, Hilda," she said, her eyes reddening. "The lump was malignant."

I was shivering. Glenn gently tucked the blanket around my shoulders and kissed me on the forehead.

"You just rest now," Nancy continued gently. "We'll talk later."

I couldn't stop shaking.

Dr. Ray had been forthright in explaining his concern about the mammogram the Friday before. The small, calcified, star-shaped spot was "worrisome." I'd gone by Nancy's office on the way home from Dr. Ray's and borrowed a medical text on breast cancer. After only a few minutes of reading the section on mammograms, I felt sure mine was more than "worrisome."

Thank God medical practices for breast cancer have changed over the last few decades. Not long ago, when a woman was put to sleep for a biopsy, she didn't know whether she would wake up with breasts or not. If the biopsy showed a malignancy, the doctor would do a mastectomy while the woman was still under anesthesia. One surgery, one anesthesia. Very straight-forward and simple. Simple, that is, except for the woman who had to accept, in the same devastating nano-second, both life-threatening cancer *and* a caved-in chest where full breasts had been. Breasts that had been a part of her since she was a budding preteen, breasts that had made love and fed babies, breasts that were the essence of her femininity.

When faced with cancer, some patients freeze, withdraw, and are unable to make decisions. I followed the opposite path. Even though, in the back of my mind, I'd clung to the hope that I was wrong, from the initial conversation with Dr. Ray, I acted on the assumption that I had cancer. I became intensely focused and completely in charge. All emotions were shelved so as not to get in my way. Every cell in my body aligned, united to save my life. Within forty-eight hours of the mammogram, I received, by over-night delivery, the most recent medical text available on breast cancer. Just off the press by less than a month, it contained all the latest information. I devoured the book. My brain fired rapidly and was instantly able to understand and remember even the most complicated and difficult information. Information far out of my field that normally would have sunk in only after laborious study. Far more than just taking in information, however, I was able to make instant connections and conclusions. Absolutely everything in me focused on one thing: survival. I tuned in to minor nuances. I read people's body language and tone of voice without effort. I was hypervigilant.

As I lay there on the gurney after the biopsy, however, the anesthesia fogged the mind of that vigilant, intelligent, energetic, and articulate woman I'd been just hours earlier. Everything was murky and mixed-up. Disoriented and bewildered, I tried to sort out all the decisions ahead of me— mastectomy versus breast-conserving lumpectomy, chemotherapy, radiation—all the things I'd already explored, but couldn't seem to remember. Where was the woman I'd been just a few hours ago? The focused, in-charge, clear-thinking professional who'd reported for the biopsy this morning?

The anesthesia was not completely done with me, however, and mercifully took me to blankness once again.

I stretched my aching back as I got up from the table where I'd just completed a bone scan. The cool tile floor felt good beneath my bare feet. It had been two days since the devastating news of the biopsy. Those two days had been filled with tests: lab work, MRIs, x-rays, CAT scans, bone scans. So far, all had come back ok. For most of the day, I'd been in the basement of the hospital where nuclear medicine is invariably located. I hadn't seen the late afternoon shadows or heard the rain-storm brewing outside. I waited for the last bone scan to be read, and then I would be finished. I felt good, strong, ready to move on to the next step.

I'd been in my most professional, in-charge mode all day as I engaged with lab techs, with radiology techs, and most especially with Dr. Ray, who informed me of the results as soon as he read each film and scan.

I'd made my decision to have a lumpectomy and radiation instead of a mastectomy. I only wished I could roll back the calendar and lose some weight. Guilt about my body had followed me since my diagnosis. I knew that breast cancer was more likely to occur in women who were obese. Now I really understood what *morbidly* obese meant! But I'd grown used to all kinds of guilt around the issue of my weight, and besides, there was nothing I could do to change the past, so I set my weight concerns aside as best I could. Overall, my frame-of-mind was good, upbeat, almost victorious, as Dr. Ray came in to discuss the bone scan.

My mood quickly changed, however, as he spoke. "We need to take a closer look at part of this last scan," he said. "There's a hot spot on your leg. It could be that the cancer has already traveled to your bone. I admit it's worrisome."

Worrisome! That word again!

On the outside, I remained calm. In control. An objective doctor seeking more information as if I were simply an interested colleague. But, on the inside, I was a frightened patient being sucked into a black pit. No woman ever dies from breast cancer in her *breast*. Only as it metastasizes to other parts of the body does it claim its victim. If metastasis had already happened, my chances of living to see my kids through college had just been narrowed dramatically.

I listened intently and nodded mechanically but heard very little after "worrisome." The blackness pulled me deeper and deeper into a place I'd never been.

"May I go to the ladies' room before the next scan?" I calmly asked.

I slowly and deliberately walked into the bathroom, removed my soiled panties, wrapped them in paper towels, and placed them in the waste can. After washing up, I went back into the nuclear medicine area and lay on the table, holding very still so as not to shatter into pieces.

The "hot spot" turned out <u>not</u> to be cancer, but only a still-healing cracked ankle that I'd injured several months earlier. It was nothing, and yet it had pushed me over the emotional edge.

I dressed slowly and deliberately, careful not to leave any part of me in the dressing room.

"Please take me home, Glenn."

He put his arms around me, and walked me to the car, protecting me from the storm with his overcoat. He said little as he drove us home, but he kept one hand on mine.

It was only 6:30 pm when we got home, but we went directly upstairs to our bedroom. He helped me undress, put me to bed, and lay beside me, gently wrapping me in his arms. My dear, sweet, unbelievably perceptive Glenn knew how fragile I was and held me together when I could no longer do so myself.

"Talk to me, Hilda." He softly stroked my hair. "I'm here, and you're safe."

Haltingly, and with few words, I told him about the bone scan.

Then the sobs came. I couldn't stop. The sobbing quickly turned to a tortured, guttural moan. The moan of an injured animal, unable to help himself.

"Talk to me," he said again. "Tell me what you're feeling."

"I don't know. It feels like I've lost something. Something important."

"What? What have you lost?"

"I don't know, but it's something important, and I'll never get it back." My moans grew louder. I kept repeating over and over, "It's gone, and I'll never get it back." I was grief-stricken over the loss of something I couldn't name.

I was glad both our children were away at college and didn't have to hear their mother's torment. Sometime in the late night hours, I fell asleep, exhausted, wrapped in Glenn's strong body.

When I awakened the next morning, still cradled in his arms, I knew what I'd lost. Sometime in the night, while I slept, it had formed in my mind, and I knew. I'd lost the only identity I'd ever known. I began to cry again, this time a sad, quiet cry.

Even though I'd known in my head that I couldn't control everything that happened to me, I hadn't known it on a gut level. That sense of control—the idea that if I just worked hard enough and smart enough and accomplished enough I could stop bad things from happening—was deeply ingrained.

Cancer could destroy me, and I couldn't stop it. For all my intellect, my ability, my driving ambition, here was something that was out of my control. I was left with nothing. And yet...I still existed. To my complete surprise, I still existed. All that I identified as me—intelligence, hard work, accomplishments—controlled nothing in this void. *But I was still present*! The essence of me, that core that had nothing to do with competence or intelligence or control was...just *was*. I just was.

That morning in 1988, a full ten years before I began tackling my binge eating problem, marked an awakening of self and laid the groundwork for later healing. I didn't know it at the time, but cancer allowed one of the most dangerous traits I possessed to be exposed as the double-edged sword it was. That trait was my need to control everything in my life, and frequently in the lives of those I loved. I had to do everything myself, do it now, and do it perfectly. In many ways, that trait had served me well, but the intense sense of responsibility for self and for others was a tremendous load to carry.

I entered my most intense control mode as I battled cancer and made decisions concerning chemotherapy. I investigated cutting edge treatments, spoke with researchers, and insisted on aggressive chemotherapy. All synapses were firing, and I couldn't turn them off. The truth was, I didn't want to! The intensity with which I battled cancer spilled over into every part of my life, and I felt more alive than I ever had.

I was both blessed and cursed by an intensity of mind and body that pushed me to find the best treatment available for my particular cancer. It was that same intensity that led me to push myself unmercifully in my practice during that time.

I worked full-time through my chemotherapy and drove myself even harder through the radiation treatment that followed. During radiation, I worked at my office straight through from eight am until two pm every day. Glenn picked me up each day at two, and I ate a sandwich as he drove me the two hours to Birmingham, where I received radiation treatment at the University Medical Center there. After completing each radiation session, we drove back in the evening, arriving home after dark. I went straight to bed, rising the next morning to do the exact same thing again. This went on five days a week for six weeks.

Not only was I working every weekday (in a hot wig, I might add), but I was more conscientious than ever. After all, the dental practice was *my* responsibility. I put on my most confident, professional face and made sure that everyone around me was comfortable with my leadership. I was more obsessed than usual that I be in perfect control of my practice, my patients, and my life. I cringe when I think about that year. What in God's name was I trying to prove?

I was like a champion race horse, fast and often the winner, but I rarely recognized the finish line. I loved the rush of the intensity with which I lived, but the driving personal demands that accompanied that intensity robbed me of the pleasure of the win.

2001

I hunched over the unconscious body of my infant grandson. I pressed my lips over his tiny nose and mouth and I tried to give him breath. My own breathing came short and shallow. The vise around my chest clamped down.

Minutes earlier, in my living room, I'd tried in vain to lose myself in needlework. I'd felt off balance and unable to concentrate ever since the 9/11 Twin Towers' tragedy three months earlier. I'd been lost in a fog of anxiety and depression shared by the whole country.

I'd just re-threaded my embroidery needle when my granddaughters, Mary and Jennifer, ages ten and eight, came rushing into my house, both shouting at once. Their terrified eyes told me more than their words.

"Aaron can't breathe!"

"Mama can't get him to breathe!"

Glenn and I jumped up and bolted out the door and across the deck that separated our house from our daughter's.

Karen, carrying Aaron, rushed across the deck toward me.

"He choked! He choked!" Her voice was high, desperate, yet somehow calm. Her pleading words were distant and almost foreign to me. One look at my daughter's face, though, and the words became clear.

Just as Karen thrust her child into my arms, his eyes rolled back, and he went limp. Aaron had passed out. All the molecules in my body lined up, and I was totally calm and in charge.

I kicked the deck's picnic bench out of the way and laid Aaron on the table.

"Call 911," I told her.

"Jennifer's dialing now!" she said.

"Go talk to them," I said. Then low and steady, "It'll be ok."

Karen took a shaky breath and ran the twenty feet to the phone just inside her door.

I was already on autopilot, doing what had to be done.

Tilt head back slightly.

Check for obstruction.

Aaron became the CPR doll I had worked on every year for the last twenty-four years. He even looked like that doll, with his round, nearly bald head, and his rubber-like arms and legs flayed out to the sides.

Cover mouth and nose with your mouth.

Give two short puffs of air.

They didn't go in.

I had less than four minutes to save Aaron.

Re-tilting his head, I tried breathing for him again.

Still, it didn't work.

Turn infant face down, head lower than body.

Five blows to the back between the shoulder blades, to dislodge the object.

Nothing came out.

I quickly turned him over and laid him on his back again.

Find hand position. Two fingers above top of sternum.

Five chest thrusts.

I was sure he would revive any moment.

I stayed focused. Calm.

Five back blows. Five chest thrusts. Two puffs of air. Over and over again.

Voices faded in and out around me. Mostly Karen's.

"Mom, is he breathing yet?"

I think Glenn answered her.

She was crying quietly, but I could hear her silent screams.

Through it all, she stayed on the phone. With EMS. Obediently answering their questions. Same questions. Same answers. Over and over.

"Honeydew! A piece of frozen honeydew."

Five back blows.

"He's just turned one year."

Five chest thrusts.

"Yes," said Karen, "my mom knows CPR. She's already doing that!"

Two puffs of air.

"Hurry! Please! He's dying!"

Busy work. That's what they're doing with her. Just keeping her busy and on the line.

Is that what I'm doing? Just busy work? Busywork as Aaron dies?

Time slowly warped, bending back on itself, to that Christmas forty-four years earlier when another life had been in my hands. Mom's life. And the lives of my brother and sisters. Dad's shadow stood beside me, haunting me. Taunting me. *Do you ever really do what's needed, Hilda? Or are you just lucky? You always think you're in control. That you can fix things.*

I shook off the ghost.

Back blows. Chest thrusts. Puffs of air.

Aaron didn't look so much like the practice doll anymore. With each blow, his lifeless arms and legs still bounced up like rubber, but that rubber had changed color. I tried to ignore the steadily-darkening purple of his skin and the coolness of his face as I covered his nose and lips with my mouth.

That fruit should be out. This cannot be happening.

My hands and arms kept going while my mind struggled to understand.

Maybe my blows and thrusts are not hard enough.

They were hard enough in dental school. "You don't have to break a rib, Hilda!" my short skinny practice partner had complained after I nearly knocked the breath out of him.

He turned to the guys nearby, "Don't mess with this girl. She's got power."

Even though he was joking, I turned red. Still, I had to do it right. Being only one of two females in the class meant that everything I did had to be perfect. I had to stay in control. I couldn't, I wouldn't, allow myself any mistakes. Mistakes were not forgiven.

I know I'm doing this right. Why isn't it coming out? Maybe I'm afraid. That's it. I'm afraid to strike hard enough. This time it doesn't matter if I break a rib. This time it's the real thing.

With the next several sets of back blows, I hit hard. Really hard.

My dad could hit hard. I wish he had hit me that night. Beat me. Smashed my face. Broken my nose again. Cut my throat. I deserved it. I should have hidden that knife. I had prayed that night, *Oh please, God, let him pass out. Let Dad stop breathing and die.*

Oh please, God, let Aaron wake up. Let him start breathing and live.

Back blows. Chest thrusts. Puffs of air.

Do it right. Be strong. Don't fail. Don't kill Aaron. Don't kill Mom.

"He's so blue!" I could hear the fear in Glenn's voice.

We both understood that time was running out.

It's almost over now. A few more seconds. I'll keep trying, but in time I'll hand my dead grandson over to my daughter, who will continue to weep and beg me to save her child. It's almost over. And I can't control it.

"You can't fix everything," Glenn had told me on more than one occasion.

"We don't always need you on your white horse, Hilda," my younger sister, Dene, had said.

A gurgle. Oh God, I've heard that gurgle before. When Glenn's dad died, I heard that gurgle. My mother called it the death rattle.

Another gurgle. And another! Small bubbles were coming out of his nose and mouth now.

Two more back blows and out came the most magnificent, slimy green bit of food I've ever seen! A tiny gasp followed. I blew two small puffs of air in to help him refill his tiny lungs. This time he took them in and slowly opened his eyes.

EMS arrived within minutes after Aaron starting breathing. We took him to the hospital in the ambulance so he could be thoroughly examined. X-rays showed nothing lodged in the lungs and no broken ribs, which surprised me. We later got a copy of the transcript and were shocked to discover that the EMTs had arrived within six minutes of receiving the call. It had seemed like an eternity!

Laryngeal spasms. That's why the fruit had not dislodged sooner. "Our worst nightmare when a child is choking," the doctor said. "This is one lucky kid."

Apparently, the cold fruit had frozen the larynx, which then clamped down *above* where the object was. So no amount of thrusts could expel it. My warm breath, however, helped melt the fruit enough for the larynx to relax. My thrusts could finally expel the fruit. Aaron could finally get air.

I went away after that. Not physically away. In fact, for weeks I didn't go anywhere. I refused to leave the house for fear I would be away from my family just when I was needed. *What if I had not been home that day?*

I took only very quick showers. *What if I had been in the tub and precious moments had been lost?* I became obsessed with my responsibility for the safety of my family. I went over and over my CPR skills. I made index cards of key points and posted them all around the house, including the bathroom so I could review them there. No, I didn't go away physically, but emotionally I was holed up in some distant canyon.

The sound of Judge Judy's voice in the den pulled me from a deep, heavy sleep. I squinted against the bright light coming through the window and glanced over at the clock. *3:00 pm?* For months I had been getting out of bed at first light, even though I had usually not gone to sleep until two or three am. How could it possibly be 3:00 in the afternoon?

As I reached with my right hand to throw the covers off, I flinched. A dull, tingling pain shot down my right arm. I rolled to the left and swung my legs off the side of the bed and stood up. *Whoa!* The muscles in my lower back were tight, trying to spasm. My breath caught and I sat back down.

After a few deep breaths, I dragged my aching body to the shower, but I couldn't bend and stretch enough even to bathe properly. After drying off as best I could, I went to my dressing room. I stepped into my panties, but they were tight and binding. Nothing fit except my old medical scrubs. *Why are they hanging in my closet*? Even after retiring from my practice, I would sometimes wear them around the house because they were loose and comfortable, but I had packed them away after losing so much weight.

What have I done? But I knew. I knew what I'd done.

I walked back into the bathroom and stepped on the scales: 251 pounds. I'd gained almost 50 pounds in the three months since Aaron's choking incident.

I returned to the bedroom and sat on the edge of the bed trying to sort things out. I didn't know what to make of it all. I thought hard. Memories of the last few months were a blur. I had dissociated before, but not like this, not this deep. This time, terror replaced the shame that I usually suffered after a severe and lengthy binge.

Where has my attention been focused? Slowly, things came back to me. Usually, when stress hit, I obsessed over work and put in longer than normal hours, staying late to rearrange files and reorganize my dental office. But I'd retired from my dental practice, so I couldn't bury myself there. Instead, I had found ways to *create* work for myself. Volunteering to organize tax information for others, I wound up handling *eight* different tax returns!

As always, everything I did had to be just so. I must have made a thousand lists. And I created spreadsheets for everything. I wouldn't pencil in some minor change on a work sheet, but rather did a whole new spreadsheet. The amount of paper and number of print cartridges I went through was staggering. I must have sacrificed an entire forest in those few months.

I lived on four or five hours of sleep a night. Glenn would coax me, "Come on to bed, honey. That can wait 'til morning."

"Just a little longer. I'll be there in a few minutes."

But the few minutes turned into a few hours. Glenn was asleep long before I came to bed, so he had no idea how little sleep I was getting. He saw me overworking, but knew I frequently did that in the middle of, or just after, some stressful event.

But no one—not Glenn, not my sisters, not my friends, not even I—was aware of what else I was doing. I was bingeing. Big time.

This episode had sneaked up on me and had been massive. I was terrified. This was serious, and I knew it could happen again and again without warning. I knew from the pain I felt in my body that I couldn't do this many more times. I was getting too old.

I finally found the courage to call for Glenn.

"Well, it's about time, sleepy head. I kept peeking in at you, but..."

As he entered the room, he stopped mid-sentence. One look at my face and he knew. He sat on the bed beside me and wrapped me in his arms. I laid my head against his shoulder, crying softly. A long time passed before I spoke.

"I was gone. This time I was really gone."

"I'm sorry. I'm sorry I didn't see what was happening."

"I'm scared."

I had been able to lose myself in binges on many occasions. All those blank pages in my journals proved that. I had become a master at dissociating. I could go about my daily life with an unmatched intensity. Everyone saw an efficient, highly successful wife, mother, and dentist. But I wasn't even present. I watched dispassionately as someone else lived my life. I was somewhere off in a corner in the fetal position. I was bingeing.

But this time felt different. Had I gone further away? Was it worse because I didn't have the external structure of my practice to balance against? Or did I just better comprehend what I had done this time?

Within a week, I was back in Patricia's office. Before she could even shut the door to her office, I burst into tears. She led me to the recliner where I always sat. She sat opposite me on the blue loveseat.

I sobbed as I told her about Aaron. I was overcome with a feeling of helplessness. He had lived, but even doing all that I could, he might *not* have. He could easily have died if the fruit had not begun to melt in time, if I had not been trained, if I had not been home, if, if, if... His living or dying seemed dependent on chance. I was tortured by my inability to ensure the safety of my family. Waves of anxiety washed over me.

When Patricia took a Kleenex for herself, I remembered that she had a toddler at home and another child on the way. She handed me the box, and took a deep breath before speaking.

"It would be natural for anyone to feel the way you do. And to still hurt. But, because of your family history, it is inevitable that you feel devastated. It will take awhile for you to regroup. Be gentle with yourself. When you were young, at a time when you should have been deciding whether to wear the green dress or the red plaid skirt, you had to make life and death decisions for yourself and your family. You felt responsible for fixing all that went on in your home. That kind of programming doesn't just go away. "

We talked for a long time about my overdeveloped sense of control and responsibility. About half way through the session, my thoughts returned to a conversation my older sister and I'd had at my cottage several months earlier. I shared it with Patricia:

Brenda and I had settled in for the day in two new leather recliners I had just bought for the cottage. A fire crackled in the fireplace. Our animated conversation slowed and became a comfortable silence.

"I want to ask you something," Brenda began slowly. "You always remember so much more than I do about the really dangerous times at home. When we talked at my house about that Christmas-time in the project when Dad had the butcher knife at Mom's throat, I realized that I sometimes have blanks and struggle to remember details. It's afterward that I remember the most. I wonder why that is."

I didn't tell her what I was thinking that day. I'd been working hard on letting go of some of the anger I felt toward Brenda. There was no reason to hurt her feelings. It wasn't her fault I still harbored some ill will toward her. After all, she had been a child too. My anger was, in fact, grounded in the very thing she spoke of now. My mind thought what I didn't allow myself to say: *It's no wonder you don't remember the crises. You were, more often than not, in a closet or under the stairs, hiding.* I couldn't get past her leaving me to stand between Dad and Mom, or between Dad and one of the other children. She was older, even if it was only by two years. I was angry because she invariably left me to bear the brunt of Dad's rage.

I just gave a sort of I-don't-know shrug. She continued.

"We never talk about what happened *afterward.* And those are the times I remember the most, what I hated the most. I hated how Dad would be so syrupy and fake-loving. How he would pull us all up into the bed to read the Bible and talk about rewriting it."

I remembered none of what she talked about. But ask me about the moment of the crisis, and I could tell you where everyone sat and exactly what everyone said and did.

"What do you remember about what happened next that Christmas?" She asked me.

"What do you mean by 'next'?"

"I mean after Dad passed out. And the next day."

"Gosh, I don't remember. Why?"

"Because that's what's so vivid to me," she said. "We needed to get out of that house, but Mom was frozen. She was just one of us. She couldn't save us."

Then Brenda began to recite the sequence of events that followed the crisis. Events about which I had absolutely no memory. She told me how she had called a friend of the family who came and got us and drove us to our aunt's house in North Carolina. She had a horrifying memory of Mom telling her that maybe it would be better if the car just went off the mountain because then, "everything would be ok and none of us would have to worry anymore."

Brenda shifted in the leather chair and pulled the afghan tighter around her legs. "If Mom had been driving, I'm convinced we would have just become headlines: *Mother and Five Children Dead after Driver Loses Control of Car.*"

She remembered arriving at Uncle John and Aunt Ivy's house at daybreak, exactly where we'd all slept in their house, how mad Uncle John was at Dad, everything. Brenda's memory of the terror of the night before may have been sketchier than mine, but when it came to the next day and the weeks that followed, she remembered every detail.

I, on the other-hand, had no memory of the long trip up to North Carolina. No memory of those days or weeks we stayed there. No memory of where I slept or what I did. My only memory of the visit (and I'm not sure it even happened at that particular time) was of Aunt Ivy's kitchen. She always had cookies in a cookie jar on the counter by the window that overlooked the hill where we played. I kept sneaking into the house to get cookies to eat. I would peek out the window to be sure no one saw me. But my aunt caught me. I thought she was outside, but she apparently had come in to use the bathroom. Surprise and guilt, and her prediction stayed with me: "Child, you're going to be as big as a barn if you keep eating the way you do."

Even after Brenda and I talked, I still had not put the pieces together. But somehow, telling Patricia about it, allowed me to see it all more clearly. In a crisis, I was unbeatable. I was super-aware of the importance of making the right decisions, of being at the right place at the right time, of interceding or not, of choosing to fight or to stand still. Heavy burdens for a young girl. So, when the immediate crisis was over, I retreated into the safety of a dissociative binge.

That was when my older sister took up the watch. That was when she called for help and got us out of the house. Her instinct to escape a crisis had kept us alive just as surely as my leadership during the immediate emergency had. We both escaped—just at different times and in different ways. As I related the story to Patricia, I understood the role we each had played. In that moment, all my anger toward Brenda simply dissolved. She had not left me any more than I had left her. We were both just surviving.

Patricia helped me to understand that I should be grateful for my past binges. "Who knows how you would have coped if you had not had food to anesthetize the pain, if you had not had the binge to hide in."

Near the end of the session I was able to verbalize my real fear. "But what if I don't come out of it the next time? What if Glenn were to die, or something like that, and I get lost in another binge and just never come back? I felt so far away this time. What if I die out there in la-la land?"

"But you did come back. You stayed gone as long as you needed to, and then you came back. And you will come back the next time, too."

"I'm not afraid to die. I'm really not. But I want to be present for my death. And I want to be present for my life. I'm just so tired. I look at people like Glenn. He doesn't struggle with life the way I do. He's such a noble human being." I paused as the import of what I'd just said sank in. "I would just like to feel that I have a little nobility before I die. I'm so tired of the struggle."

"There are all kinds of nobility," Patricia answered softly. "There is nobility in the struggle too."

I went back home, resolved to be kinder to myself. Resolved to appreciate the nobility in my struggle with living. And with my binge eating. My bingeing stopped and, within several months, my weight dropped back down to 202. I couldn't help but hope that maybe this time, with my new insight, I would even be able to avoid bingeing at the barrier that had remained for so long.

But as my weight dropped, the nightmares started again. And once again, each time I woke up, I was left with a strong feeling that I must gain the weight back. I resolved to get to the bottom of that fleeting thought. It no longer mattered that much to me that I weigh below 200, but *why* that particular weight was a barrier mattered a great deal. I wanted to know what was happening and why.

I did a relaxation meditation each night before going to bed and each morning upon arising. *Find a way to understand, Hilda. Why do those dreams always come on the heels of losing weight?*

I dropped below 200 pounds, enlisting Glenn's help so I wouldn't "get lost" in food. But the nightmares worsened as they always had, and the urgency to regain the weight grew stronger. And my hunt for whatever it was that connected that weight and nightmares grew more intense.

After several weeks of this, I woke up one morning weeping. As always, Glenn encouraged me to talk.

Through the sobs, all I could say was, "I feel so weak...so...so *frail*."

"Why would you feel frail?" He made me keep going.

"I don't know. I'm just not strong like I used to be, and it makes me feel awful."

"Hilda, you walk every day; you lift weights. You are far more fit than you used to be. Why on earth would you feel *weak*er?"

It was true. I *was* healthier and stronger than I had ever been. And suddenly it came to me! I understood why I felt weaker and why my psyche wanted me to weigh more. I had a very powerful reason for wanting to stay fat. And it was all bound up in that intense feeling of responsibility that I wrestled with. My strongly-held image of myself as a very large person was essential: I needed to be really big in order to protect myself and those I loved!

I knew *logically*, of course, that I was far stronger and more able to defend myself when I was leaner, but my childhood experiences dictated otherwise. As a young child, it was clear to me that big people (especially big adult men) had all the power over others. Dad was bigger and stronger and could easily overpower the rest of us. That distorted thinking became the basic building block of my attitude about weight.

I had taken on the role of protector early in life. The role was constantly reinforced by my mom. *You are my Rock of Gibraltar, Hilda. What would I do without you?* From a very early age, I stood between Dad and his victim, whether that victim was Mom or one of my siblings. It was *my* bed Mom retreated to for safety and comfort after a night of violence, even when I was only seven or eight years old.

The sense of being responsible for the safety of my family was instilled in me very early and was a huge influence in the formation of my personality. I remember, even as a very young child, daydreaming about getting bigger and stronger.

What was indeed true in childhood—*Big adults have physical power over small children*—was taken to the extreme. The distortion became: *The bigger I am, the stronger and more powerful I am.*

And, because of my intense sense of responsibility, the lie got even bigger. *I am responsible for the safety and well-being of those I love, and if I don't do everything possible to stay big enough to protect them, then I am an evil, irresponsible, and selfish person.*

Is it any wonder that my unconscious would do everything possible to keep me fat? My nightmares were always about my inability to help those I loved, most especially my children. It all made so much sense now.

Weakness in any form was unacceptable and any show of vulnerability was a sure sign of weakness. I became fiercely independent and self-sufficient, unwilling to allow myself the luxury of needing help and comfort. And the more threatened my "fat" status became—200 pounds was apparently the magic number for me—the more unwilling I was to let down my guard.

But no one can live under that kind of pressure for long, so the binge beast had come to my rescue. He taught me early that when the battle got to be too much, when I absolutely had to rest, there was a way, a way I could keep my identity intact. I could dissociate from my "strong" body and seek the comfort I could no longer do without in *his* arms. I could go to that sweet, soft, unconscious land of the binge and find solace. Until I returned from that place, I didn't have to feel anything. Not pain, not weakness, and, most of all, not responsibility.

I now could easily see that my body image as a very large person was no longer of value. My fat couldn't make me feel strong and safe any more. But that knowledge left me with an even bigger problem. Once I understood that my fat couldn't insulate me from danger, there was no going back to that haven. I now felt more unsafe and unprotected than ever before.

For months, I could find no solace, no place to hide from my ever-present sense of both responsibility and vulnerability. A new kind of dread and fear set in. I called Patricia. "I can't, and won't, go back to where I was; but I can't bear to live this way either. I don't know what I want anymore."

"Yes, you do," she responded. "You just want to feel safe."

And so I set out to find safety. If a large body couldn't protect me and make me able to protect others, then what could? I exercised relentlessly, working hard on strength training. I delved deeper into positive self-talk and strength imagery. I watched movies about strong women who could, and did, protect themselves and their loved ones. My DVD library expanded to include *Alien, Terminator II, Matrix, G.I. Jane, Enough*. I read biographies of strong women. But nothing helped.

As a last resort, I enrolled in an intensive eight-week self-defense class offered by the Police Academy. I hoped that this would do what all the strength training, self-talk and imagery, books, and movies had failed to do.

For weeks, the seven of us in the class learned smart ways to stay out of danger and how to look less like a potential victim, how to get away quickly and safely, and how to disable an attacker with smart moves. We practiced good defensive posture in order to maintain our balance (rule #1: do not go down if at all possible). We practiced how to circle and kick if we were taken to the ground (rule #2: do not get pinned if at all possible). We went over how to block and parry, how to kick and hammer fist, how to heel-stomp and shin-scrape. And on and on.

I was beginning to think this just might be what I'd been looking for. But then the last day of class came. The "final exam."

In the back of the room was all the gear we had used in practice: helmets, face guards, skin protectors, gloves.

Joe, our main teacher, instructed us, "Put it all on, ladies. Tonight you get to show me and Pete what you've learned."

He then explained that he would lead us, one at a time, with our eyes closed, into another room where he would position us in front of a fake ATM machine. We could not open our eyes until we were "attacked." Once attacked, we would try to "escape" off the mat and tag Joe, at which time we would be "safe" and officially pass the test.

Joe left the room while we geared up.

"If Joe is the one to lead us out," Tiffany, one of two tiny high school seniors who were taking the class before heading off to college, said, "then you know who the attacker is going to be—Pete!"

We all groaned. Pete was 6'6" and the most muscular man I'd ever seen. I would never want to meet him in a dark alley! The attacker always wore full body protection so we could hit and kick as hard as we wanted and there was no danger of him being injured. But with full gear (Jason mask and all), Pete was a very scary man!

As we put on our gear, we encouraged each other. We had already been exposed to several "attacks," so we ran through the different ways we could be grabbed: by the arm, by a choke-hold, by trying to pin our arms down from the back. We reminded each other of the seven basic strategies of defense: brace for balance, head butt, elbow strike, hammer fist to the groin, knee strike, shin scrape, heel stomp.

I felt confident, but Tiffany and Tara looked pale.

"We've done it all in class before," I assured them. "Remember what they've drilled into us: DON'T PANIC. Just shift from one technique to another until the attacker releases," I authoritatively quoted from the manual.

Both blonde ponytails bobbed, but they didn't look convinced. I was glad for them that I had drawn the first position.

Joe came back into the room. "Hilda, you're up."

As he led me into the room and up onto the mat, I mentally rehearsed the routine that I'd practiced so many times. *Brace for balance, head-butt, elbow-strike....*

He placed my right hand on the paper ATM machine pasted to the wall. I barely touched the wall when, suddenly and forcefully, in one split second, I was in the air! High above Pete's head! He had grabbed me from behind, pinning my arms, and—all in one motion—had lifted me up and over his head! We both went down on the mat (too late for rule #1!) and he immediately pinned me face down onto the mat (rule #2 out the window). I was terrified, as if Pete were a real assailant. I was totally unprepared for this maneuver, which was his goal, of course. Everything was a blur! And I was frozen.

From the sidelines, I heard Joe shout, "Yell, Hilda! Fight!"

I heard myself, weakly at first and then loud and angry, "STOP! HELP!"

My adrenaline was pumping and I began to resist. But what to do? Nothing seemed to focus in my brain.

Joe again. "Get that right arm out straight; left arm in close." ROLL, ROLL!" he shouted.

I could get no leverage, but I kept going. *Get your elbow up! Just get him off you!*

I felt helpless. I was tiring and thought I had nothing left in me. After what seemed an eternity, I felt Pete let up a little and I managed to roll him off me and climb on all fours off the mat. I stood and ran toward Joe.

I felt Joe's hands on my wrists as he said, "Whoa! I'm not the attacker." I then realized I was beating Joe's chest with my fists while still screaming *STOP! STOP!*

Embarrassed, I walked off to the side and waited for Joe to bring in Pete's next victim. I knew that neither I, nor any of the other women in that class, could *really* get away from Pete. I felt *less* safe than I had before the class had begun.

After the class was over, all the other women talked about how much more empowered they felt. Not me! I knew my only hope of escape was for my assailant to be exceedingly stupid! I might out-smart him, but I could never out-fight a muscular 6'6" testosterone-pumping machine.

I cried for weeks. I felt lost and ungrounded, unable to hold one thought for long.

I was trying to express how I felt to Glenn one day, but with little success, mainly because I couldn't pin down exactly what I was feeling.

"I feel so helpless and exposed. Like somebody has died. Like I'm in mourning or something."

"Maybe you *are* mourning, Hilda," Glenn said, pulling me in close. "Maybe you're mourning the human condition of being vulnerable."

Everything shifted ever so slightly as the thought sunk in. It was one of those moments that we rarely get in real life. I stopped crying and repeated to myself: *The human condition of being vulnerable*.

That was it! That was absolutely it!

The obvious became clear. We human beings are indeed fragile and unsafe. We can only protect ourselves to a limited degree. And it's all relative. I may be weaker than a six-foot 50-year-old, but he is weaker than his 25-year-old counterpart. And any of us can be struck by lightning or a car tomorrow. Or get cancer. Or choke on a piece of frozen fruit.

The world may not be as unsafe as I saw it as a child, but the bottom line is that to be human is to be vulnerable and, of course, ultimately mortal. I had to mourn that human condition of vulnerability before I could move forward. It was a very sad time for me, not only because I was reminded of how fragile life is, but also because I realized how much of my energy had been spent fighting that notion my whole life.

Yet there was a comfort in accepting how little I could do, a comfort in no longer having to constantly protect myself and those dear to me. I was tired, and for the first time in my life, I didn't have to be a warrior anymore. I could finally lay down the last of my armor and rest.

Chapter Ten

Relax the Grip: Letting Go

"We must be willing to let go of the life we planned, so as to accept the life that is waiting for us."

Joseph Campbell

1994

I sat across the desk from Dr. Ames, waiting for his response to my unusual request. His distinguished graying temples, deeply tanned skin, and kind face reminded me of Robert Young in the role of Dr. Marcus Welby.

"Are you sure about this, Hilda? This is a pretty drastic step you want to take," he said. He reminded me that I'd been cancer-free for the last six years.

I knew I was being aggressive. My cancer had been small and I'd done well with chemotherapy and radiation. And even though I'd had five breast biopsies done on suspicious lesions since the original cancer, each one had been benign. But I was confidant and clear-headed as I sat and listened to all the reasons that I should not do what I was determined to do.

My friend, Nancy, was no longer practicing medicine, so I'd turned to Dr. Ames, a respected surgeon at M.D. Anderson Hospital in Houston, hoping he would do what many doctors and most patients would consider unthinkable: elective double mastectomies.

Six years earlier, when I'd chosen to have a lumpectomy, leaving my breasts intact, I hadn't counted on the worry caused by new suspicious areas constantly popping up, or the inevitable biopsies that followed. With each biopsy, a new scar appeared on my mammogram, making diagnosis increasingly difficult. Concern that a new cancer might be lurking unseen behind one of those scars kept me constantly watchful.

Even though I stayed vigilant, I was no longer really troubled about that *original* cancer. I knew I'd done all that I could, and felt confident about my decisions to have a lumpectomy, radiation, and aggressive chemotherapy. What I was worried about, however, was the possibility of a *new* cancer. Statistically, nothing puts a woman at more risk for a new, second breast cancer than already having *had* breast cancer. The factors that contributed to my cancer in the first place—genetics, nutrition, exposure to DDT as a child, as well as all the unknown risks—were still a part of my history, so the chance of getting a new cancer was very high and very real. After each of the last two biopsies, I'd resolved to be rid of the worry by having elective double mastectomies. But first I'd wanted to lose some weight. The story of my life.

My son, Tim, had just had twin boys. I now had four grandchildren, all born within the last three years. Head-over-heels in love with each one of them, I couldn't bear the thought of not sharing their lives. The day after the twins, Steven and Michael, were born, I'd found a suspicious lump in my breast. It turned out to be benign, but it hastened my decision to go ahead with elective mastectomies, even before I could lose weight.

So when Dr. Ames asked if I was sure, I answered without hesitation, "I am absolutely positive."

"Ok, then, I'll do the surgery. Given your history, it's not really an unreasonable precaution."

I exhaled with relief.

"But, I want you to wait a month," he said. "That will give you time to fully reconsider your decision."

"Thank you."

"Have you thought about reconstruction?" he asked. "We could coordinate with a cosmetic surgeon and he could start implants that same day."

"Maybe later, but right now I just want to have the mastectomies." I was not enthusiastic about implants and simply didn't have the energy to look in-depth at other options.

I walked out of Dr. Ames's office, feeling good about my decision. Now I had a month to prepare.

During that month, I concentrated on my health. I ate well, exercised, and got plenty of sleep. The most important thing I did, however, was to create and practice a special visualization.

Many women say that cancer brings a sense that their bodies have betrayed them, and they just want their breasts gone. One woman even told me, "The thought of them being on my body one more minute was almost unbearable. I wanted to cut them off myself!"

I didn't feel that way at all. I wanted to show appreciation for my breasts and all that they had been to me. After all, breasts are among the most life-giving parts of a woman's body. They are a part of how we make love; they are how we feed and nurture our babies; they are an integral part of who we are. In order for me to live fully, they had to be sacrificed. A sacrifice that felt like the ultimate life-giving act. But I didn't want to lose the essential feminine part of me that they represented, or to let them be taken away without proper reverence.

Decades earlier, a television special on kids with leukemia had first introduced me to visualization as a healing adjunct to cancer treatment. All the children in the study got the same chemotherapy protocol, but half were coached in the use of visualization. They were told to imagine Pac Man traveling through their bodies, gobbling up the cancer cells. The children who were taught this technique not only had better remission rates than those who had not, but also had fewer side effects from treatment and fared better emotionally.[1] When I'd had chemotherapy, I'd used my own version of their visualization. It had been very effective, keeping side effects down and my spirits up. This time, however, I was looking for a different kind of effect.

In that month before my mastectomies, I began each day in the same way. While still lying in bed, I'd take in several long, slow breaths, then imagine a beautiful soft blue and pink mist above and around me. I thought of the mist as all that was good and beautiful in the world. As I breathed in, I brought all that goodness and beauty into my body. I imagined it streaming into my breasts and gently capturing all the feminine and life-giving qualities residing there. As I exhaled, the essence of my breasts were gently disseminated to the rest of my body, into my hair, my skin, my toes, all of me.

With a second breath, I again took in the mist, but as I exhaled this time, I released stress and anxiety. I let go of any ill will and resentment toward myself and others.

I linked a third breath to thoughts of waking up from surgery warm and comfortable, refreshed and peaceful. I continued this special three-breath meditation for ten or fifteen minutes, and then ended with a simple, silent *Thank you*.

Together, Glenn and I celebrated my breasts. We talked about the joy they had brought us: the stolen pleasure the first time he touched them, the weight and feel of them in his hands underwater the night we went skinny dipping, and the pride we both felt as I nursed our babies. We mourned their coming loss, but at the same time, celebrated our unbreakable bond, a bond that was far more than beautiful breasts or memories of what had been.

In the last few minutes before surgery, my body and mind felt calm and rested. I was ready. No second thoughts, no regrets, only eagerness to be free of the fear of a second cancer. As the nurse anesthetist administered the anesthesia, she commented on my steady heart-rate and blood pressure. I smiled and said a silent final good-bye to my breasts.

I opened my eyes to a pretty young Hispanic nurse adjusting a warm blanket around my feet. There was no struggling out of anesthesia this time. I felt comfortably warm, alert, and peacefully happy. The young nurse noticed that I was awake and smiled. She walked to the head of the gurney and put her small hand on my shoulder. In a lyrical accent, she said, "Hello, Mrs. Lee, my name is Gigi, and I'm going to take good care of you."

What started as a tiny secret smile on my lips quickly grew to a wide grin and a soft giggle. What a perfect moment! My mom had been the last person I'd seen before Glenn and I left Alabama a few days earlier to come to Houston. She had put *her* hand on my shoulder and said, "I can't come with you, Hilda, but I'll be with you in spirit. I'll be looking over your shoulder, taking good care of you."

Mom's and nurse Gigi's words were similar, but what made me smile was the fact that everyone in the family called my mother "G.G." for "great-grandmother."

The warm blanket around me was nothing compared to the warmth I suddenly felt toward Mom and her desire to take care of me. Mom loved me. She did the best she could even though she hadn't been able to help any of us kids feel safe and nurtured when we needed it the most. It's ironic that Mom was always the one to nurse people when they were sick or dying: her mother, her siblings (she outlived them all), even neighbors. Mom's mantra was, "All I ever wanted was to be a wife and mother." But somehow she was too dependent herself to take care of those most dependent on her—her own children. She wanted to. She really wanted to. And at this moment, with nurse Gigi's hand on my shoulder, I felt peaceful and grateful toward my mom and her noble struggle to be the mother she so longingly wanted to be.

I once heard someone jokingly refer to the *pie chart of guilt*. How much responsibility and blame do we assign to ourselves and how much to various others in our lives? I'd spent a great deal of energy trying to accurately divide the pie chart of our family's misery. When I was very young, it was easy—I blamed myself. I claimed the whole pie. As I grew up, however, I began to understand that it was not all my fault. That's when I assigned Dad an ever-larger wedge of the pie chart. Eventually, though, I began to appreciate parts of him that had been invisible to me as a child: his intelligence, his perseverance, even his Irish charm during periods of sobriety. He was indeed a thief—he had stolen my childhood—but I eventually became aware that the demons that pursued him were kin to those that haunted me and my siblings.

And so, as I reduced Dad's slice of the pie chart of guilt, I'd expanded Mom's. Over the last few years, my resentment toward her had grown as I tried to figure out how much of the family pain I could assign to her. I could no longer excuse what she did or didn't do, and say she was just a victim, even though that was true enough. She was still the adult in our family, and therefore responsible for us. I resented her dependency, her silent passivity, her unwillingness and/or inability to leave and take us out of that house. I resented having to take on adult responsibilities at the age of ten. And yet, by understanding that she did her best, and by looking at my own mistakes as a parent, I could no longer blame her without empathy.

I'd been thrashing around in this quandary for years, trying to get the blame just right; thrashing around, that is, until I realized what a complete and utter waste of energy the whole futile process was! *It's time to quit assigning guilt! It's time to tear up the pie chart! Life is what it is.*

We're not just the sum total of what we do right and what we do wrong. Our actions count and count a lot, but so does what's in our hearts. My parents' motives counted. Dad did love us and wanted us to have a good life, but he was driven by something none of us would ever fully understand. How did he draw *his* pie chart? He failed to protect us—was, in fact, the biggest threat to us—but I have to believe that he hated that part of himself as much as we did. Mom loved us, and wanted more than anything to be a good mother and, at least in many ways, simply couldn't be. Was that her fault? Dad's fault? Their parents' fault? It didn't matter anymore. Now, from my own safe place, I could accept the caring that I know they held in their hearts, but were unable to deliver.

And so, as young Gigi tucked in my blanket and placed her hand on my shoulder, I felt assured in some cosmic way that Mom, the *other* "Gigi," was like this sweet angel. I was engulfed in a tenderness from—and for—my mom that I'd never felt before.

My visualization was complete. So much had changed in the month since I'd approached Dr. Ames to do my mastectomies. My whole body now carried the femininity of my breasts. I'd accepted the maternal part of my mother that had eluded me for most of my life, and I would never again be burdened with the fear of another cancer in my breasts.

"Is everything all right?" Gigi asked, not knowing what to make of my unexpected joy, especially given the circumstances.

"Oh yes, everything is perfectly all right," I said.

I placed both hands on my now flat chest and felt whole for the first time in a very long time.

2002

I stopped sweeping the expansive back deck for a moment and, for the last time, watched it rain on the lake. It was one of those odd days when the sun shines, yet rain falls. The lake shimmered in the sun as raindrops broke what had been a smooth and glassy surface only minutes earlier. The lake was less than fifty yards away, yet rain fell only over the water, not on our house or the green lawn that sloped down to the water's edge where tall, silvery-plumed pampas grass gently swayed. I'd seen isolated rain over the lake many times in the twenty years since we'd built this house, but it never ceased to amaze me.

Later this day, Glenn and I would give the keys to our house to the new owners. I was surprised at how much easier it was to leave our home than it had been to part with my beloved practice. Turning my dental practice over to my partner, Lisa, was one of the most difficult things I'd ever done. I'd started the practice right out of dental school in 1977, and it had grown from just one dental assistant and myself to a thriving practice of four dentists and twenty staff members.

I loved both patients and staff. We celebrated together through graduations, weddings, and births. Once a teen-age patient drove his new car—an old rusted bright orange Vega— by my office from the used car lot; he wanted me to admire his new wheels. More than once, new parents had brought their babies by on the way home from the hospital.

My patients, staff, and I also mourned together. I cried with new widows, wept for middle-aged men who died from heart attacks, mourned young women's lives cut short by breast and uterine cancer, and watched patients and staff care for their elderly parents. I suffered along with families torn apart by abuse, divorce, Alzheimer's, and death.

Likewise, my patients and staff saw me through the graduations and marriages of my children, the births of my grandchildren, breast cancer, several surgeries, and the near death of two of my grandsons. We also laughed loud and often; the door on our staff refrigerator was covered with jokes and cartoons patients and staff had brought in. Patients shared funny incidents, photos of family vacations, even clippings from a new rose bush or potted plants. Many brought in their favorite foods, from bar-b-que and brownies to sausage biscuits. Once a patient delivered her favorite German cake to my house on Christmas Day because I had met her at my office on Christmas Eve to solve a dental problem.

I was connected to my patients and staff in a way that made leaving difficult. I'd tried cutting back my hours and working part-time for a while, but I still worried and fretted over the practice full-time. After returning from my stay at the center in North Carolina, I realized I simply couldn't make all the necessary life changes from within the practice that I so loved. I decided that my highly productive career had made for a highly stressful life, and I would have to make a choice between my health and my practice. I chose health. Lisa and I spent years making the transition a positive experience for patients and staff, but it was still with a great sense of loss that I finally stepped aside in 2001 in order to save my life.

I pulled myself from thoughts of the practice and resumed my sweeping. This home in Lacey's Spring had been our dream: a house on fifty acres, overlooking our own private lake. In our vision of what would happen in that dream, Tim and Karen would come home from college and share stories of collegiate life as they drank hot chocolate by a fire; that dream never came true since both rarely made it home at the same time and, when they did, they were soon off with their friends. We'd dreamed weddings would take place on the expansive deck of our home; both our children, however, wanted church weddings. We envisioned grandchildren freely playing ball on the back lawn while Glenn and I watched from rockers on the porch; that rarely happened since the parents were afraid the kids would drown in the lake and we seldom had time to rock.

We were sure that both our children would build their own dream houses on this dream property and then their children would do the same, and then...well, you get the picture. Tim and his wife had no desire to live so far from the city. And, while Karen and Brian and their kids did live on the property for a short while, it was not *their* dream, not *their* future. When Karen hesitantly broached the subject of selling it and getting a smaller place, more suited to their lifestyle, I felt a relief I'd not expected, a surprising relief to let go of a vision I'd held too tightly, a vision of not only mine and Glenn's future, but that of our kids as well.

Our property in Lacey's Spring had served us well for many years, but while we were not looking, it had become a burden. A burden we were holding onto because we connected it so intensely with home and family. But the reality was that the yard had become too much yard, the house too much house, and frankly it never looked like I'd imagined anyway—bushes died, flowers went to seed, and something always needed repairing. Once Karen spoke up, I quickly realized the property had become our version of Walton's Mountain, and none of us, most especially me, fit the Walton image!

Once we resolved to sell and move, the process of weeding out began. For two long months we made decisions about what to keep, what to give away, and what to throw out. Any old family furniture the kids didn't want, along with Corning Ware, Norman Rockwell prints, assorted tools, clothes and shoes, and glittery prom formals more than filled a moving van from Goodwill. Over a thousand books—I counted them— went to the library, schools, and used book stores. Did I really need my ninth-grade Latin book anymore? Several trips to the dump in a pick-up truck unloaded old bent bikes that hadn't been ridden for decades, broken weed-eaters, pink drapes from a previous house, and on and on. The pleasure of stripping down our possessions was intoxicating!

By the time we moved, we had only essentials and a few truly cherished items. Once I could not have imagined leaving our dream home; now I couldn't imagine staying. I was getting good at this letting go!

I could also let go of the last of the excess weight that had defined me for such a long time. After the incident with Aaron and the subsequent realization that having a large body no longer served to keep me safe, I began a short daily visualization specifically to release the fat that I no longer needed. I visualized that all the strength and power that I had once thought resided in my large body could now be filtered into my core.

It was a simple exercise, but the fat seemed to melt away. According to Jung and other psychologists, imagery is the language of the subconscious, and the more we use the language of imagery, the more we can connect to our subconscious, to primal patterns ingrained deep within us.[2] The use of imagery helped me to let go of deeply ingrained learned patterns that no longer served me.

Over a period of several months, I'd steadily and comfortably moved down from the 200 pound mark that had been such a barrier for me. I now weighed 185, a weight that felt "right" to me, a weight at which I moved easily and felt comfortable in my clothes. As I had learned more and more about myself in my struggle with binge eating, I had gained a confidence that I would know when I reached where my body instinctively wanted and needed to be. That weight, by the way, that was at the very top of the BMI "overweight" category, which happened to be (as I mentioned earlier in the book) the "healthiest" weight according to recent studies.

The next year, when I returned to Duke for a follow-up visit, I was delighted to reconnect with Betty, a friend I'd met there when I'd first come in 1998. Betty had been a veteran of dealing with binge eating disorder longer than I, and was somewhat of a mentor figure for me. Athletic and agile, she virtually bounded everywhere she went. She was the picture of an active, healthy forty-year old. Her short, dark hair framed a kind face, and her ready smile drew others to her.

The week had been full for both of us, but after lunch on Friday we met in my room. Tired from our morning workout, but happy to finally have some free time, we settled on opposite ends of the sofa, kicked off our shoes, and began what would be an all-afternoon visit.

Light chit-chat soon turned serious as we discussed relapse. She shared some of her major relapses with me, and I told her of the huge binge that had followed the episode with Aaron. We struggled to find the right words for how major relapses affected us.

I read her the poem I'd written a few days after I'd come out of that last dissociative binge. It expressed how I felt better than any other words I could find:

> *My silent screams could not be heard.*
> *No sweet smile of child nor touch of lover's hand,*
> *Could reach me in the darkness of the binge.*
>
> *I did not choose that ungodly place,*
> *But there was a comfort in that space.*
> *The pain was somehow lessened by the void*
> *In that darkness of the binge.*
>
> *Did Satan suck me into Hell*
> *From which I could not see or hear or feel?*
> *Was it punishment for being weak and frail of heart?*
> *Or was it mercy on God's part?*
>
> *And yet my fingers, numb before, now ache and burn*
> *From my terrored grasp around the cord*
> *The golden cord.*
> *The cord that led the ancients from the labyrinth's depths*
> *Now guides me back to humankind*
> *From that darkness of the binge.*

Betty's eyes teared. "Sometimes it feels like both punishment and mercy."

We sat quietly for a few minutes. Then Betty spoke again. "Relapses can be rough." she said. "Used to, when things were going along smoothly, I'd feel hopeful, like I'd never slip again. But now I know better; I know I'm only an emotional crisis away from faltering. Not completely devastating, can't-seem-to-move, all-out failure, but faltering nonetheless."

She paused to take a sip of her soda. "But, you know something? I make a lot of progress when I falter. Just like you did after this last big set-back. One step back, two steps forward. That's why now, instead of *relapses*, I call them *prolapses*. Like a folding forward rather than a falling backward."

Prolapse, not relapse. Hmm. What we call things matter, and the word *prolapse* was an ideal image for what had happened to me over the last several years. I thought about the pattern of my progress. I'd always made the most *physical* progress when it was smooth-sailing. That's when I'd lost weight, reinforced good habits, stabilized. But the dark times led to the most *emotional* progress, which opened up new possibilities for me. I was then able to surge forward with new insights, making strides that were impossible before.

"Those falling backward times do seem to help me understand myself better," I said.

"I think it's because that's when we uncover obstacles we didn't know were there. Then we can deal with them head-on."

"Yeah, but the cost of that progress is high. It takes me a while to pick myself up again. I felt pretty beat up this last time," I said.

"Maybe we'll eventually learn to fall without hurting ourselves, like my friend," Betty said.

I didn't know what she was talking about and must have looked puzzled.

"I haven't told you about my friend Carlie? The one with cerebral palsy?" she said. Betty sat her soda down on the coffee table in front of us and settled back on the sofa, tucking one leg under the other. She told me how she and Carlie often went places together and how well her friend got around on crutches.

"Most of the time I forget she's handicapped," Betty said. "But one day, we went somewhere and had to go down a steep flight of stairs. I held my breath as I watched her maneuver down the stairs ahead of me. When we were both at the bottom, I asked her if she wasn't afraid she would fall. Without hesitation, she answered that she *did* fall sometimes, but that one of the first things her parents taught her when she was a very little girl on crutches was how to fall. 'You shouldn't be afraid of falling,' they'd told her, 'or your life will be very limited.' Carlie had to learn to fall without hurting herself. She apparently learned to roll when she fell, to use her shoulders and hips to minimize the damage."

Then Betty said something that helped me put meaning to recent changes in my life. "Sometimes we just have to let go and roll with the fall. That letting go is part of learning to fall safely."

I'd been letting go of a lot of burdens in the last few years and, for the most part, the process had been liberating, even exhilarating. Occasionally, though, it had been a terrifying free fall, especially when I tumbled into a major binge. I don't know if the time will come when I never binge again, but now I have a safer image, one of rolling *with* the fall instead of fighting against it. That image eased my anxieties and made the fear of future binges less frightening.

After dinner that evening, I sat in my room alone and quietly revisited what all I'd released over the course of my recovery. I'd let go of a lot of things: a house that no longer suited me; burdensome possessions that I no longer used; my beloved dental practice that had brought much joy but also stress; breasts that had to be sacrificed in order to save my life; even the weight that I no longer needed for protection from a world I'd seen as unsafe. But all these *things* were nothing compared to the intangibles that I'd let go. Intangibles like resentment toward my parents and my circumstances; perfectionism and all-or-nothing thinking; shame associated with bingeing; a crushing sense of responsibility. Letting go of all that armor meant a lighter load and a far better life.

One of the most important things I'd let go, however, was the idea that my binge beast was some external monster to be killed. I'd come to see him as an intricate part of *me*. An essential, powerful part of me that I'd denied. He was everything that I'd loathed and feared about myself. He was like my shadow. He still had the power to frighten me, but somehow I'd made peace with that shadow, much like I'd made peace with my inner critic, Millie. I was learning to dance with my shadow, and it was exhilarating.

The whole idea of making peace with and dancing with my shadow reminded me of a famous fresco found among ancient Greek ruins. It depicts the sport of bull-leaping, where young athletes grab the horns of the bull and leap over his back in a sort of graceful dance between man and bull.[3] When I'd first seen a photograph of that fresco, it struck me as a wonderful image of dancing with my inner beast—dangerous, yet graceful and exhilarating.

I'd looked up a photograph of the fresco while reading a book called *Bull from the Sea* by Mary Renault. Betty had recommended it when I told her how I was using the myth of Theseus and the Minotaur in the book I was writing on my experience with binge eating. Renault was fascinated by the possibility that this fresco and other ancient ruins found on the island of Crete were the origins of the famous myth. In her book, she looks, through fictional eyes, at history and archeology, and constructs a story of what Theseus' life and adventures *could* have been if he had been a real person instead of a mythical character.

In Renault's story, young men and women from conquered Athens are sent as tribute to Crete and are forced to become "bull-dancers" to entertain the wealthy of Crete.[4] Notably, the ancient ruins that were actually found during excavation show that the real palaces of Crete had huge courtyards surrounded by hundreds of rooms, stairwells, and workshops that make the palace look more like a convoluted town than a single building. Many historians believe these structures were the origins of the mythic labyrinth.[5]

In the fictionalized version by Renault, most of the enslaved bull-dancers live only a short time before being gored to death. Theseus, who volunteers to be one of the young slaves, eventually leads a revolt and frees the slaves. But first, he has to become part of one of the bull-dancer teams. Unlike other teams, where each acrobat works for his own safety, Theseus convinces the members of his team to become interdependent and to protect each other. Together, they become unbeatable, They even make peace with the bull, enlisting him to be a part of their team.[6]

I love this rendition of the myth. It is powerful and nuanced. And is a remarkable reflection of where my own journey has taken me. The world doesn't have to be about fighting and struggling and winning. It can also be about appreciating and cooperating and unifying. The Minotaur, half bull, half man, is strong and powerful, but real strength is found, not in killing that vigor, but in embracing it. Theseus' bull was not, in the end, an evil enemy, but rather a respected and intricate part of the team. By learning to "dance" with their bull, they had turned him into an ally. By learning to dance with my shadow, I had gained a powerful ally of my own.

After showering that evening, I stood naked in front of my full-length mirror and smiled at the body I'd once hated. *This ole body has served me well.* I looked at the body which I now loved and had a new appreciation of it. I then made a decision I hadn't expected.

I pulled at the eight or ten inches of excess skin that remained around my middle as the result of my massive weight loss. I was proud of it. It represented the hard work I'd done to become healthier, but now, suddenly, it no longer felt necessary. I was free to change it, free to release it. I was fine with the jiggling arms. I accepted the cellulite on my legs that was a part of me. I was ok with—even proud of—the scars where breasts had once been. But this loose, hanging skin suddenly felt unnatural to me. It felt like I needed to wiggle from this last cocoon. I smiled at the image. Just like that, the decision was made. I would have a tummy tuck and let go of the skin I no longer needed.

Relax the Grip: Letting Go

PART V

RETURNING HOME

Theseus emerges from the labyrinth a wiser young man. He triumphantly returns to his beloved home in Athens where he restores what was once a wasteland into a vibrant, bountiful place of plenty, overflowing with new life.

Thereafter, Theseus feels compelled to tell his story to all who will listen.

Chapter Eleven

Transformation

1997

I struggled through the frozen underbrush, crouching and bending to avoid the low-hanging trees bowed over with ice. My legs were rubber, and the cold wind invaded my lungs, making each labored breath all the more painful. My weight, nearly 300 pounds, plus the heavy coat, gloves, and clunky boots that I wore, made the uphill trek on the frozen rutted road agonizing. I was breathing hard and lagging farther and farther behind Glenn, as he clipped along almost effortlessly even though he carried a large bolt-cutter, a small ax, a flashlight, and two battery-powered lanterns.

"Are you sure this is the right way?" I called to Glenn. "Shouldn't we be there by now?"

"I'm sure this is right. But we can stop and rest," Glenn said.

Glenn's sense of direction was always good, but the hike up the road seemed longer than I remembered. "No, let's keep moving. It can't be very far." Even though I was physically spent, my excitement grew. Besides, the sooner we got to the cottage, the sooner we could get out of this cold. The lone crunch of ice breaking beneath our feet echoed all around as we trudged up the old logging road.

The snow and ice had looked good from inside the warmth of our car on the trip up. It had, in fact, provided one of the most memorable sights I'd ever seen. The sky had been clear from Alabama to Atlanta and Greenville and on past Traveler's Rest, but everything changed about half way up the mountain. Suddenly, near Caesar's Head State Park, we were surrounded by ice. Every branch of every tree dripped with ice diamonds. We had reached the frozen rime line, and entered a magnificent crystalline forest of ice. I'd never seen anything remotely like it. Sunlight danced through the frozen jewels, and the trees became giant chandeliers.

But now, walking outside in that same cold, I paid less attention to the landscape and more to my freezing, over-taxed body.

We'd made the trip, even after we knew snow and ice was a possibility. We were eager to see inside our new mountain cottage. A week earlier, through a transaction done by mail, we'd purchased the 242 acres on which the cottage sat. The abandoned house, which we both knew would most likely never be inhabitable, had been included in the sale at no additional cost. No one, except us, had given the old cottage much thought. We'd seen the building from the outside, but neither we, nor any of the realtors involved, had ever set foot inside the boarded-up cottage.

"Here's the marker we left. We're close," Glenn said. He immediately turned off the logging road and advanced through frozen bushes. I kept my head down and my arms in front of my face to shield me from the icy branches as I hurried to catch up. The sound of ice crunching ahead of me served as my guide. Suddenly, it was quiet. Glenn had stopped. I looked up. Glenn and I stared at the sight before us.

"Oh my," I said.

We never intended to buy so much land. Or spend so much money. And we certainly didn't expect to buy an old dilapidated house. We'd wanted several acres on which to build a small vacation home, but had fallen in love with this large tract of land with its pristine mountain, a lake, and several waterfalls. On the far side of the land, near the lake, were some old, run-down camp buildings. We'd been told that the volunteer fire department would be glad to burn them down, "along with an old cottage somewhere on the property," for practice drills.

When the realtor first showed us the land back in October, we'd also asked to see the cottage. He had a hard time finding it because it sat back from the logging road and was almost buried behind huge rhododendrons; so huge, in fact, that they all but hid the house. That day in October, the realtor guided us past the bushes to find the back door bolted shut, and the steep front porch steps too rotted to use. The cottage had revealed little of itself to us as we'd stood on tiptoes to look through dirty windows. Glenn said it had two bedrooms; I said there couldn't possibly be more than one. He said there was a kitchen; I saw none. He said there were stairs to some kind of attic; I said no way. He'd looked through a back window, I through a side. About the only thing we agreed on was that some furniture was stored inside the dark, ugly house. While neither of us had any real hopes of salvaging the cottage itself, we both hoped for hidden treasure inside.

Now, here we stood, a week after buying the property, with our own 242 acre mountain, twelve dilapidated camp buildings, and a house we had not even seen inside yet.

Huge rhododendrons, laden with ice, draped over the cottage. Not one board of the wood siding, not a door, not a window was visible beneath the bushes and ice. The chimney peeked above the tallest treetops and was the only hint of a house beneath.

"Let's go! Let's get inside!" I said, eager to see what we had.

"Just hold on a minute. Let's don't go rushing in," Glenn said. "We have no idea what's inside. The floor or roof may be rotted; there may be small animals in there."

"Maybe a hibernating bear!" I added, almost wishing there would be.

"We don't want to surprise—or be surprised—by whatever we *do* find." Glenn led the way as we pushed through the last of the frozen underbrush to the back door. Using the bolt cutters, he snapped the lock off the door and cautiously shined his flashlight inside.

"What can you see? Hurry up and get in so I can see too." I felt like a ten-year-old on a secret expedition into forbidden territory.

We stepped into the frozen cottage, more like a cave than a house. The ice-laden bushes that pressed up against the windows left the inside like a scene from *Dr. Zhivago*. Even though it was only mid-afternoon, little sunlight penetrated the cave.

The flashlight and battery-powered lanterns provided the only light, but we saw enough to know we'd found our treasure. We didn't know that we were about to embark on a restoration that would consume the better part of a year, or that the restoration would, in many ways, foreshadow, and even facilitate, my own personal transformation that would begin the following year.

The inside was dry and well-preserved. We entered a large L-shaped living area where a stone fireplace dominated the room. Old wicker rockers sat roughly in a semi-circle around the fireplace hearth; antique chests and rustic tables lined the walls; a wooden sofa and two matching chairs with faded cushions sat to the side; an interesting metal floor lamp stood nearby. The dining area off to the side had a long table surrounded by eight cane-back chairs. Newspapers and magazines, all dated fifteen years earlier, were strewn on a large library table which we later learned was custom built for the cottage's owner in 1925. The floors, ceilings, and even the walls were long-planked, tongue-and-groove yellow pine.

Off this large multi-purpose room we found a full kitchen, equipped with stove, refrigerator, and an antique china cabinet full of dishes. A huge porcelain sink, with plates and cups apparently left to dry on the attached drain-board, flanked one wall. Two stiff, faded dishrags hung on a wooden wall rack, and canisters filled with sugar and flour sat on the counter.

We turned and made our way down a long hall. A once-white chenille robe hung on one of the dozen or so wall hooks along the wall. Off the hall, we found *four* furnished bedrooms. Beds were made, a few items of clothing hung in a closet, and shoes sat neatly by a dresser. There were two bathrooms with beautiful porcelain sinks and big, oversized claw-foot porcelain tubs. This house was far larger, and far nicer, than either of us had guessed. Someone obviously had intended to return. Why else would shoes and clothes be left in the bedrooms, clean dishes left to drain in the kitchen sink?

A staircase fashioned from twisted rhododendron branches led to an upstairs sleeping loft where two iron bed frames and several mattresses lined the walls. In one corner sat a battered trunk. The romantic in me wanted that trunk to be full of old love letters. No such luck, of course, but hand-embroidered spreads, hand-made quilts, and a forty-eight star American flag all lay neatly folded inside.

We longed to stay and explore the drawers and cabinets packed with dishes, games, knick-knacks, and papers, but it was getting late, and we weren't sure if the roads would remain passable into the nearby town of Brevard where we had reservations for the next two nights. We'd be back tomorrow. The roads into town were icy and deserted, but we slowly made our way to the hotel where heat and a warm bath awaited us.

Over the next few months, the history of the place unfolded. I learned its history by meeting the son of the man who'd built the house, by lunching with the woman whose in-laws had been the original owners, and by spending a delightful day with the ninety-one year old who'd once been the caretaker for the cottage for fifty years.

In 1925, the president of a textile mill near Greenville, South Carolina, had bought the 242 acres to build a camp as a summer retreat for mill workers. He'd also built a summer home for himself and his family a short distance from the camp. That summer place was the cottage we now explored. After he died in 1948, the mill and all its holdings were sold to a large textile enterprise out of New York who eventually sold the camp and the cottage to the Elks Club. The family of the deceased president, however, was allowed to continue using the house as their summer retreat. They came up each year for Brevard's summer music festival. When they'd last come, in the summer of '83, the family fully expected to return the following summer, as they had for almost six decades.

But before the next summer, ownership changed again. The Elks sold the property and everything on it. The house was locked up and lay dormant until we bought it fifteen years later. We're convinced that the new owner never even *saw* the cottage. He had bought the property for the land itself just as we had done. The cottage's out-of-the-way location and overgrown surroundings had sheltered it from the elements, and from vandals. By the time we bought it, only a few of the people in the community even knew of its existence. A few of the windows had small cracks from fallen limbs, but the structure remained tight and protected.

The cottage had been refurbished in 1946 and had been preserved in that state, just waiting for us to come along and save it. Even though Glenn and I had never had any interest in restoring an old house, this cottage was worth saving. We felt as if we were stewards of the property and had a responsibility to it. Plus there was something serendipitous about it being last upgraded in 1946, the same year I was born. As I saw what could be done with the house, I think I unconsciously saw better possibilities for my own life as well.

Tarry creosote, used in years past to prevent rot, covered the outside of the wooden building, giving it a dark, ugly appearance, but that unsightly coal tar is what saved it from the elements and from the termites, somewhat a miracle in its damp environment. After a strong pressure washing and a new coat of stain, the cottage was as lovely outside as it was inside. I often compare myself to that cottage. For many years, I was buried beneath a not-so-attractive exterior, an exterior that had protected me somewhat from the "elements" of my early life, but one that could be changed when the time was right.

The questionable infrastructure had to be redone for safety and comfort: new plumbing, new electrical, central heat and air. We tore off and replaced the roof, or rather roofs (there were four layers of separate roofs that had been added over the years). Those layered, heavy roofs saved the inside of the building and its furnishings. As each layer of roof was peeled away, as the burden to the house was lessened, the contractor said he could all but hear the house breathe a sigh of relief. In the years to come, as I peeled layer upon layer from my own overburdened body and spirit, I would come to know and appreciate that same feeling of relief. And appreciate how protective my own layers had been over the years.

What to discard and what to retain always presents a challenge. I wanted the cottage to be fresh and functional, solid and safe, but I didn't want to change its basic nature. Some decisions were harder than others. I insisted, for example, that we keep the original windows with their beautiful wavy pressed-glass panes, even though they didn't seal as well as new ones would have. "That's ok," I said. "Let the cottage breathe a little. It's been tightly sealed way too long."

In the course of the many months I spent in that house, hosing down walls, scrubbing cabinets and closets, repairing and refinishing furniture, I also spent many hours in an old wicker rocking chair looking through those old distorted windows, examining what was and what could be in my own life. A quiet sadness fell over me as I watched the world through the haze of tears and wavy glass. But, somehow, those months cleansed me, prepared me for the difficult journey that would begin within a year.

Over the years, we've uncovered numerous stone walls and stone patios, even a lovely garden behind one low stone wall. We restored the garden and named it *Ruth's Garden* in honor of the woman who originally prepared it in the late '20s. Every time I think I've uncovered all there is to find, however, something new presents itself. Only last month, I found the remnants of an old stone path behind the house.

I contacted the unofficial historian from the Greenville textile mill, now in his nineties. He, and several of the old campers from the 1930s and '40s came up for lunch in the cottage after I'd completed the renovation, and shared stories of their days in camp. He then gave me a copy of the camp ledger which chronicled camp activities all the way back to its opening day in 1925. Just like my own journals helped me understand my life, those camp journals helped me reconstruct much of the history of the camp, and what life was like in those early years of the 20th Century. Within their pages, for example, I found what happened day-to-day in the years of the Great Depression when the camp provided a much needed respite from the battered world beyond.

It took almost a year to complete the renovation of that cottage and make it into our own family's retreat. The restoration not only paved the way for changes in my own life, but the process awakened a creativity in me that I never knew was there. I'd always considered my sisters to be the creative ones. I'd never been happy with my decorating skills. No matter how much I planned and worked, no house I lived in ever seemed *right* to me. The colors were never quite what I thought I'd picked; the stripes in the sofa were either too broad or too narrow; the chairs were too little, the lamps too big. But with this cottage, everything I did seemed *right*. To this day, almost twenty years later, every detail still pleases me. And to think how close the cottage came to being burned down by the fire department. Treasures are often found in the most unlikely places.

2003

I stood erect and still, arms stretched straight out to either side, as Dr. Sullivan moved around my body, drawing lines with a red marker. The next morning I would undergo surgery for the final phase of breast reconstruction, as well as an extended tummy tuck. The first phase, in which the skin and fat from my abdomen were used to form new breast mounds, had been done months earlier. Now the really tough part was about to begin. And I was having second thoughts.

I hadn't planned on so much surgery when I first went in search of the right doctor almost a year earlier. After losing so much weight, I'd decided I wanted a tummy tuck, nothing more, just a simple tuck to get rid of excess belly skin. I'd had two babies, been obese since those births, and now, in my late fifties, had very little skin elasticity left. I'd earned a tummy tuck. And I was, at first, against reconstructing my breasts. While I would have liked my breasts back, I was also perfectly comfortable *without* them. In fact, I appreciated how, in some strange way, *not* having them had helped me heal emotionally. My mastectomy scars were proof of my desire and ability to make hard, life-changing decisions, proof that I was taking charge of my own life.

I no longer needed such proof. The reason I'd first decided against reconstruction was because I didn't like what I thought were the only options available. I knew many women who'd had silicon or saline implants and were happy with them, but the idea of having a foreign substance in my body gave me an uncomfortable, almost queasy feeling. I felt awkward trying to explain this attitude. After all, I'd abused my body for years, and saline implants were pretty innocuous, but implants just weren't for me. The other standard option for breast reconstruction was a TRAM flap procedure which sacrificed abdominal muscles. That was out of the question for me. I'd worked too hard on core strength to give it up for breasts.

My search for the right surgeon and the right surgery turned up Dr. Scott Sullivan in Louisiana and a brand new procedure known as the DIEP flap. This was a microsurgery that used the fat from a tummy tuck but spared all the muscles. I was a good candidate, and my insurance would pay for it. His only concern was the esthetics around my waist. I'd lost so much weight that if he stopped at the sides (as with a typical tummy tuck), I'd be left with puckered areas at my sides, and rolls of skin still around the back of my waist. So he recommended removing the excess skin around the entire circumference of my body.

He had fully described this procedure, but I'd not understood just how much skin would be involved until I watched him draw the red marks on my body. I stood rigid, stunned as he lifted large areas of skin, and continued to draw. Finally, he finished and stood back for a final check. I was covered in red marks from my breasts to my thighs.

"Are you really going to be able to take this much off?" I asked, pointing to the area around my waist and hips.

"Absolutely," he said. "What I will be doing is much like altering a dress that's many sizes too large. Some of the fabric has to be removed. Because you've lost so much weight, your skin is now too large for the body beneath, so I'll remove part of it." He walked back to me and gently lifted several inches of excess skin. "Then, after this is gone, I'll reconnect the skin above and below." He gently tugged at the hanging skin, stretching it away from my body, and used the blunt end of the marker to retrace some of the red marks he'd just made. "See. When this is connected, it will be smooth."

I felt queasy.

"This is going to be remarkable," he said, more to himself than to me.

He was seeing what I couldn't imagine—and wasn't sure I wanted to. Dr. Sullivan, young and totally self-assured, had made me feel safe from our very first meeting, but I now needed additional reassurance.

"And you can keep me comfortable, right?" I asked.

He put the red marker down, handed me a robe, and motioned for me to sit back down on the examining table. He rolled his stool over to face me.

"Yes, I'll keep you comfortable. But please remember what I told you: you *will* need pain meds this time. *Please* take them from the beginning. It's much easier to *prevent* pain than to stop it once it's in full force."

I'd been very comfortable after the first surgery, and had needed no pain medication. While Dr. Sullivan had been a little surprised that I'd taken none, he explained that most women do quite well with that surgery. But he warned me not to underestimate the extent of this second procedure. "It'll be fairly extensive. Far more than a simple breast reconstruction or a tummy tuck."

I'd spent the last few months preparing for this second phase of surgery. I ate healthy, exercised, and stretched every day. I had a massage every other week and listened to my own music in the sessions, the same music I'd gotten permission to use during surgery. Just as with my mastectomies, however, the most important thing I did to prepare for surgery was my daily visualization. Because it had worked wonders in my chemotherapy, my mastectomies, even for the weight-loss itself, I'd become a firm believer in what my mind and body working together could do.

At least three times a week I did a full relaxation and visualization session using all I'd learned about mind/body healing over the years. My breasts had been sacrificed in order to save my life years earlier. I'd had to let them go in order to protect myself. This skin that was about to be used to restore my breasts was the symbolic residue of the bingeing that had protected my life while I was lost in the labyrinth. I had let go of bingeing in order to once more save my life. It felt like everything about my body had come full circle. It felt satisfying, complete.

I had done all I could to be prepared and felt ready for the transformation my body was about to experience. But seeing all those red marks gave me pause. What had I committed to?

After seven-and-a-half hours of surgery and literally yards of sutures, I should have been in agony. I was heavily sedated right out of surgery, but once I woke up I was alert, comfortable, and hungry for real food. Any one of the procedures Dr. Sullivan did during the surgery—final shaping of the breasts, nipple reconstruction, refining the belly with an extensive tummy tuck, and removing excess skin around my entire circumference—was enough for significant pain. Yet, with only the anti-inflammatory medication which Dr. Sullivan insisted that I take to keep the swelling down, I was totally pain-free. In fact, a warm, pleasant, tingling sensation spread throughout my body, which is how I'd envisioned any necessary discomfort. Once again, my pre-surgery visualization had come through for me.[1]

What Dr. Sullivan had been able to do was nothing short of astounding. My breasts and the whole nipple-areola complex looked so natural. *This* is what Dr. Sullivan had seen when he marked my body, and what I had been incapable of even imagining.

Four weeks after surgery, I stood in front of the full-length mirror in Parisian's dressing room and hardly recognized the woman looking back at me. *It's me! It's really me! Me in a fitted dress!* Tears blurred my vision. *I have curves! I have breasts!*

Slacks, scrubs, and sweats, all bought through mail-order, had made up the bulk of my wardrobe for more than thirty years. At my largest, even mail-order didn't carry women's clinic jackets big enough, so I'd had to buy men's jackets and have the arms shortened. Even a man's size 46 jacket wouldn't button.

When each of my two children got married, I'd had dresses tailor made for my impossible-to-fit body. The last dress I'd actually *bought* had been decades earlier—a baggy, low-waisted, size 28 from a Lane Bryant catalog.

I was at Parisians to buy a good bra. For the first time in ten years, I needed a *real* bra for *real* breasts! As I passed by the dress section on the way to the lingerie department, however, I was drawn to the beautiful outfits on display. The new styles were stunning. I immediately thought of Karen, and her girls, Mary and Jennifer. I loved to take them shopping.

I'd seen nothing in stores like these clothes, though, not since the early '60s. The idols of my youth—Elizabeth Taylor, Audrey Hepburn, Jackie Kennedy—would have been happy to wear *these* dresses. One dress in particular stood out. A straight, sleeveless, black-and-white polka-dot.

I wish Karen liked fitted clothing; this dress would look so good on her. Maybe Mary could wear it. No, the style's too mature for her. Oh, I know—how about Dene? I fingered the fabric in admiration, trying to figure out who could wear such a classic, when a saleslady about my age approached.

"Aren't the clothes beautiful this year?" she said.

I nodded. "I was just thinking how good this would look on my daughter."

"Your daughter? Why don't *you* try it on?"

My cheeks flushed. *What does this size ten know about the challenges of shopping when you're as big as I am?* Before I could leave and escape any further humiliation, the lady had already pulled out two of the dresses.

"What are you? About a 12 or 14?" she asked.

In a flash, I remembered I had lost a lot of weight. Maybe I *could* shop here now. But hardly a 12 or 14.

"I have no idea what size I wear, but definitely not *that* small," I said. "I've lost over 100 pounds and haven't shopped for a dress in decades. My guess is about an 18." I secretly dreamed of a 16. I hadn't been in a dress that small since before I'd gotten pregnant with Tim 38 years earlier, but I knew an 18 was more realistic.

She laughed. "No way are you an 18, Honey! Here, start with this 14."

I stiffened. "Thanks, but I'll try the 18." My words came out cool and flat. Maybe she was sincere, but she'd touched a nerve. How many clerks in my youth had patronized me with flattery? *That style is so slenderizing* or *My, that cut really shows your womanly figure*, or *Those vertical stripes make you look taller*. I'd learned early about subtleties and nuances. When teachers talked about underlying meanings in essays and short stories, I was way ahead of them. I got my education early.

"We don't carry an 18 in this department, but you're not going to need it," she said, seemingly unaware of my shift in tone. "Here, take this 14, along with a 16, but the 16's going to be too big." She grinned knowingly. "My name is Jan, and you and I are going to have fun today!"

Yeah, lots of fun. I took the two dresses and looked around for a dressing room near the exit, prepared for a quick escape when neither fit.

"This way," she said.

I followed obediently as she directed me toward a dressing room in the opposite direction.

I nervously entered the dressing room and pulled shut the curtain, hoping the 16 would somehow miraculously fit.

I vividly and painfully remembered the last time I'd shopped—or rather tried to shop—in a department store with "normal" sizes. The incident had occurred more than thirty years earlier, but every word of the conversation was seared into my memory:

"May I help you?" The clerk's blue hair and matronly manner were standard for the old-guard salesladies of the '70s in the South.

"I need a dress for a friend's wedding next month. It's been a while since I bought anything and I'm not sure of my size. I've gained a little weight."

"Oh, Sweetie, we won't have anything in here to fit you. Have you tried one of the fat-lady stores?"

There had been nothing subtle about *that* clerk. That had been the last time I shopped for myself in a local clothing store until today. The incident plagued my mind as I undressed.

I slipped the size 16 over my head, fully expecting to have to struggle into it. Instead, it slid on effortlessly, hanging loose about my body. Jan was right—it was too large!

I tried the 14 and it fit perfectly. It clung to my waist and hips, accenting curves I hadn't seen or felt since my teens.

As I stepped outside the dressing room, Jan was waiting for me.

"Look at me," I said, tears flowing unabashedly. I held my arms out from my sides and turned so she could see me from all sides. "Look at me! I'm in a size 14!"

"Here, I thought you might need this," Jan said as she smiled and handed me a tissue box. She motioned for me to turn again. "You're lovely."

I never did get to the lingerie department that day, didn't buy the bra I'd come for. I wanted to try on everything in my size. I didn't, but I did buy a red and yellow sundress and that pretty polka-dot one.

Chapter Twelve

Full Circle: Coming Home

The frozen blueberries I scatter on top of my Honey Oat cereal quickly frost over as I pour cold milk into the bowl. I peel a small speckled banana, stir Splenda into my cup of hot tea, and place everything on a wooden tray, next to a caddy of colored pencils and the beautiful new coloring book I found hidden under my pajamas last night—another of Glenn's "shiny objects." Glenn knows how much I've been enjoying those wonderful adult coloring books that hit the market a few years ago. This one, a collection of intricate kaleidoscope patterns, is especially unique.

Still wearing my pajamas, I carry the tray onto the screened-in porch, perched high above the ground like a treehouse. I am especially drawn to the porch when, like today, it rains. Glenn left early to visit his brother in Chattanooga, so I have the whole day to myself. I sit in the wicker rocker that has been on this porch since long before we restored the cottage more than ten years ago.

My sense of the present fills me with pleasure: the ping of rain on the metal roof, the muted bark of a distant dog; a soft spring breeze through the pines; the musty smell of the wet earth; the beautiful pink and white rhododendron in full bloom. *Now this is the way to spend a rainy day*.

I eat slowly, savoring each delicious blueberry. So different from how I used to eat. After finishing my tea, I climb into the hammock, taking my new coloring book and pencils with me.

There is nothing I have to do, no place I have to be except right here, right now.

A few Christmases ago, Karen gave me a pink and beige lap blanket she had woven. It quickly became my favorite throw. I pull it up over my legs and snuggle deep into the hammock. Lying here, gently swaying, listening to the soft rain, I am totally present. I have learned to be mindful of life, whether in joy or pain; I have learned to be present for my life, while eating or while making love. I know that developing awareness in my everyday living is one of the great blessings that resulted from my having to deal with binge eating.

There are, in fact, many such blessings. Healing and recovery is about so much more than the mere absence of bingeing. How different I am from the person I was a decade ago. Physically and emotionally I am healthier and more comfortable in my body and mind than I ever dreamed possible. But with these physical and emotional changes, another more subtle transformation occurred in my spirit. I slowly but steadily, let go of my old world view and embraced a new one.

Even my vocabulary has changed. When I was first diagnosed with binge eating disorder, I'd envisioned myself *battling* a monstrous binge beast. I'd *hated* that beast and had resolved to *brutally kill* him. Slowly, as I began to understand that the binge beast had carried me through some very tough times, times when I might not have survived without him, I softened toward him. I came to appreciate him and what he'd done for me.

Where my operative words used to be *battle* and *struggle*, now they are *appreciate* and *accept*. Where I had once wanted to *win*, I now want to *cooperate*. Where I had once sought *victory*, I now seek *peace*. I have always known how to fight. But I had to learn how to dance. Dance with my shadow.

I love this cottage in the mountains of North Carolina. Restoring it in 1997 preceded the beginning of my own personal transformation less than a year later. So in late 2003, when Glenn and I moved into the cottage and made it our permanent residence, it felt like I was coming home. I had come full circle

It has stopped raining, but I remain snuggled in the comfortable hammock. I pick out a bright red pencil and begin coloring one of the kaleidoscopes in my new book.

When we decided to move into the cottage, I made another decision as well. I enrolled in graduate school in nearby Asheville. I wanted to learn more about the science and psychology behind binge eating, wanted to improve my writing skills, wanted to be challenged in a classroom full of bright young minds. And I am so glad I did.

One of the reading assignments for the first class I took was a book called *Centering: In Pottery, Poetry, and the Person.* It was an old book, published in the mid 1960s. I had never heard of it, but that book put words to a subtle change in my life that I'd previously been unable to articulate.

One Sunday afternoon I went to the university's library. It had a copy of the book, but it was listed as restricted and couldn't be taken from the building, so I planned to spend the afternoon there reading it.

I signed for the book and went upstairs. From what I could tell, I was the only person on the entire floor. When I was in undergraduate school, students filled the library on Sunday afternoon but now, with computers and on-line research, college libraries are often deserted, even on week-ends.

I settled in a corner at one of those wonderful library tables you only find in older universities. The wooden kind with surfaces all worn smooth from use. The chairs are comfortable in spite of the fact that they are wooden and straight-backed. Their contours fit the body as no other chairs do, and somehow they always feel warm, like someone just sat in them for hours, even if the library just opened.

I love old books. They have their own unique history. The oils from all the hands that have touched them give them a matte look, a matte feel. As I hold them and read them, I am a part of their ongoing history. Even the musty smell of old books fills me with pleasure.

I especially loved the look and feel of that tiny little hardback I held that Sunday afternoon. Its cover was faded and worn, its binding frayed, its spine broken many decades earlier. Its musty odor, familiar.

I opened the book. The very first line took my breath away:

> _Centering_: _that act which precedes all others on the potter's wheel. The bringing of the clay into a spinning, unwobbling pivot, which will then be free to take innumerable shapes as potter and clay press against each other. The firm, tender, sensitive pressure which yields as much as it asserts._[1]

That simple definition encapsulates a subtle change that has taken place in me over the last few years, a change that I'd never found words for but had slowly leaned into. The transformation in all areas of my life has been remarkable. I didn't kill my love of food; I simply transformed what I ate from something that destroys into something that nourishes. I didn't deny my appetite, but instead discovered it, finding joy in food, as well as in other aspects of my life. I've transformed impulsiveness into joyous spontaneity, stubbornness into perseverance, and released perfectionism to embrace the pleasure of excellence. But what happened to me while I was in the midst of my struggle was more than these transformations. I had been out-of-pivot, and was finding a new center.

My life made a subtle, yet powerful shift because I unconsciously accepted the need for a *firm, tender, sensitive pressure which yields as much as it asserts.* Too much yielding and the clay—uncontained and uncontrolled—flies apart, collapses. Too much exertion and the clay is crushed. Throughout my life, I'd been heavy on *assertion*—will-power, self-reliance, impossible perfectionism—and only *yielded* when I acquiesced and collapsed in that far-away land of dissociative bingeing. As a result of that lack of *centering*, my life had repeatedly collapsed, just as the clay collapses when too much exertion is applied.

As both potter and clay, I've been able to find that new center. I like this person who can both yield and assert, this person who is now free to just *be*.

I look at the colors of my kaleidoscope, pleased with what I've created. The blues and reds and golds I've chosen bring to mind my sister's kaleidoscope. The one I took apart as a child. I'd so wanted to find the source of its beauty, and was broken-hearted when all I found inside were bits and pieces of broken glass. It has taken me a lifetime to understand that the beautiful patterns of a kaleidoscope are because of, and not in spite of, the fractured shards inside. And that the shadows dancing 'round the edges add to the depth and beauty.

Likewise, I had only seen the broken bits and pieces of my own life, and thought they made my life ugly. But I am who I am because of *all* my experiences. The good and the bad, the joyful as well the painful. Throughout my life, I'd yearned for something extraordinary, something exquisitely beautiful, and now I have discovered that beauty deep within myself and in the life that surrounds me.

I can now gently lean into life with a sense of nobility that has come from within my struggles. My journey through the labyrinth has brought me home to myself.

<u>Note from Author</u>:

I am committed to sharing the message that there is hope and recovery for those lost in the labyrinth of binge eating. If you found this book useful, please help me spread the word by telling others, and by posting information about this book on Facebook and other social media. Thank you for helping me to help others.

SEND COMMENTS ON THIS BOOK TO THE AUTHOR:

hildadlee@gmail.com

CHAPTER NOTES

Introduction

1. American Psychiatric Association, *Diagnostic and Statistical Manual of Mental Disorders-V* (Washington, D.C.: American Psychiatric Association, 2013).

2. James I. Hudson, Eva Hiripi, Harrison G. Pope, Jr, and Ronald C. Kessler, "The prevalence and correlates of eating disorders in the National Comorbidity Survey Replication," *Biological Psychiatry* 61 (Feb 2007), 348-358.

3. American Psychiatric Association, *Diagnostic and Statistical Manual of Mental Disorders-IV* (Washington, D.C.: American Psychiatric Association, 1994). In 1994, the *DSM-IV* did not recognize binge eating disorder (BED) as a separate and distinct eating disorder, but rather listed it in Appendix B using the catch-all category of "eating disorder not otherwise specified" and recommended it for further study. In 2013 DSM-V, however, BED was recognized in its own category as a separate eating disorder.

Chapter 1

1. American Psychiatric Association, *Diagnostic and Statistical Manual of Mental Disorders-V* (Washington, D.C.: American Psychiatric Association, 2013). When the author attended Duke's weight-loss center in 1998, the criteria for binge eating disorder was bingeing at least two days a week for six months (which is how it appeared in the DSM-IV at that time), but the criteria was changed to once a week over a three month period in the 2013 *DSM-V* so the information in the narrative was changed to fit the updated 2013 criteria.

2.   Information on binge eating was first presented to the author of this book at Duke's Diet and Fitness Center in1998 as part of her treatment there. The information was actually presented over the course of three binge classes, but is compressed here for convenience and aesthetics. The author's subsequent research on her own and while in graduate school further clarified and expanded her knowledge on the subject. For readers interested in a more in-depth look at specific topics related to binge eating, please refer to the resources listed at the end of these chapter notes.

Chapter 2

1. Ulrike Schmidt, "Risk factors for eating disorders," in *Eating Disorders and Obesity*, ed. Christopher G. Fairburn and Kelly D. Brownell (New York: The Guilford Press, 2002), 247-250.

2. Daniel Goldman, *Emotional Intelligence* (New York: Bantam Books, 1995), 17.

3. Rick Glantz, *Managing Cravings*, (Battle Ground, Washington: Rhea Jacobson Management, 2001), cassette.

4. *Ibid*.

5. Mary Dallman, *Online Early Edition of the Proceedings of the National Academy of Sciences* 100, no. 20 (2003).

6. *Ibid.*

7. For more information, read works of self psychologists, such as Heinz Kohut, *The Restoration of the Self* (New York: International University Press, 1977).

Chapter 3

1. Centers for Disease Control and Prevention. www.cdc.gov (accessed July 26, 2015).

2. Rachel Christine, "The average woman vs. the average model," *Thoughtful Women,* March 19, 2014 (accessed July 26, 2015).

3. Ann Oldenburg, "Miss Indiana Mekayla Diehl praised for 'normal' body at Miss USA show," *USA Today*, June 2014, (accessed Aug 31, 2015).

4. *MODE*, June, 2000.

5. *Largesse, The Network for Size Esteem*, 2002, "Facts And figures about dieting and weight loss," http://www.largesse.net/ (accessed August 26, 2005).

6. Kathy Kater, "Transforming the harmful Effects of Thin Privilege and Weight Stigma by Promoting Health Instead of Size." Presented at the Binge Eating Disorder Association (BEDA) annual conference on Nov 6, 2015.

7. Janet Polivy and C. Peter Herman, Dieting and binging: A casual analysis," *American Psychologist* 40, no. 2, (Feb 1985), 193-201; Glenn Waller, "The psychology of binge eating," in *Eating Disorder and Obesity*, ed. Christopher G. Fairburn and Kelly D. Brownell (New York: The Guilford Press, 2002), 98-102.

8. *Ibid.*

9. *Ibid.*

10. Walter H. Kaye, "Central nervous system neurotransmitter activity in anorexia and bulimia nervosa," in *Eating Disorders and Obesity*, ed. Christopher G. Fairburn and Kelly D. Brownell (New York: The Guilford Press, 2002), 272-277; Christopher G. Fairburn and Paul Harrison, "Eating disorders," *The Lancet* 361, no. 9355 (Feb 2003), 407-425.

11. Janet Polivy and C. Peter Herman, "Experimental studies of dieting," in *Eating Disorders and Obesity*, ed. Christopher G. Fairburn and Kelly D. Brownell (New York: The Guilford Press, 2002), 84-87.

Chapter 4

1. Azeem Ghorayshi, "Too big to gulp: How our sodas got so huge," *Mother Jones*, June 25, 2012, http://www.motherjones.com/media/2012/06/supersize-biggest-sodas-mcdonalds-big-gulp-chart (accessed July 26. 2015); Robert Klara, "The tall, cold tale of the big gulp," *Adweek*, Feb. 16, 2015, http://www.adweek.com/news/advertising-branding/tall-cold-tale-big-gulp-162960 (accessed July 26. 2015); Kelly D. Brownell and Katherine Battle Horgen, *Food Fight* (New York: McGraw-Hill Companies, 2004).

2. Kelly D. Brownell and Katherine Battle Horgen, *Food Fight* (New York: McGraw-Hill Companies, 2004).

3. "Sin City eatery features 8,000 calorie burger," *ABC News.go.com*, 2015. http://abcnews.go.com/Health/video/sin-city-eatery-features-8000-calorie-burger-14715607 (accessed July 26, 2015).

4. "Obesity and overweight," Centers for Disease Control and Prevention, Jan 21, 2014,

http://www.cdc.gov/nchs/fastats/obesity-overweight.htm (accessed July 26, 2015).

5.   Kelly D. Brownell, *PBS*, www.pbs.org/ (accessed August 23, 2005).

6.   Michael Strober and Cynthia M. Bulik, "Genetic epidemiology of eating disorders," in *Eating Disorders and Obesity*, ed. Christopher G. Fairburn and Kelly D. Brownell (New York: The Guilford Press, 2002), 238-242.

7.   Kendler, K.S., C. McClean., M. Neal, R. Kessler, A. Heath and L. Eaves, "The genetic epidemiology of bulimia nervosa," *American Journal of Psychiatry* 148 (December 1991), 1627-1637.

8. James F. List and Joel F. Habener, "Defective melanocortin 4 Receptors in hyperphagia and morbid obesity," *The New England Journal of Medicine* 348, no. 12 (March 20 2003), 1160-1163; Michael Strober and Cynthia M. Bulik, "Genetic epidemiology of eating disorders," in *Eating Disorders and Obesity*, ed. Christopher G. Fairburn and Kelly D. Brownell (New York: The Guilford Press, 2002), 238-242; C.M. Bulik, P.F. Sullivan , and K.S. Kendler, "Heritability of binge-eating and broadly defined bulimia nervosa." *Biological Psychiatry*, 44, no. 12 (Dec 15, 1998), 1210-1218; T. Reichborn-Kjennerul, C.M. Bulik, K. Tambs, and J.R. Harris. "Genetics and environmental influences on binge eating in the absence of compensatory behaviors: A population-based twin study." *International Journal of Eating Disorders,* 35, no. 3 (Nov, 2004), 307-314.

9. Sadaf Farooqi et al, "Clinical spectrum of obesity and mutations in the melanocortin 4 receptor gene," *The New England Journal of Medicine* 148 (March 20, 2003), 1085-1095.

10. Ruth Branson et al, "Binge eating as a major phenotype of melanocortin 4 receptor gene mutations," *The New England Journal of Medicine* 348 (March 20, 2003), 1096-1103.

11. James F. List and Joel F. Habener, "Defective melanocortin 4 Receptors in hyperphagia and morbid obesity," *The New England Journal of Medicine* 348, no. 12 (March 20, 2003), 1160-1163.

12. George A. Bray, *Contemporary Diagnosis and Management of Obesity* (Newtown, PA: Handbooks in Health Care, 1998).

13. National Institute of Health, "Binge eating disorder (Publication No. 04-3589)," *WIN: Weight Control Information Network*, September 2004, http://win.niddk.nih.gov/publications/binge.htm. (accessed February 12, 2006).

14. R.A. Grucza, T.R. Przybeck, and C.R. Cloninger, "Prevalence and correlates of binge eating disorder in a community sample," *Comprehensive Psychiatry* 48, no. 2 (March-April 2007), 124-131.

15. Cynthia M. Bulik, "Anxiety, depression, and eating disorders," in *Eating Disorders and Obesity*, ed. Christopher G. Fairburn and Kelly D. Brownell (New York: The Guilford Press, 2002), 193-198.

16. Cynthia M. Bulik, "Binge Eating Disorder and Psychiatric Comorbidity." Presented at the BEDA annual conference, Nov. 6, 2015.

17. National Center of Addiction & Substance Abuse at Columbia University (CASA). "Food for thought: Substance

abuse and eating disorders" (Dec 2003). New York: CASA.

18. Michael Strober and Cynthia M. Bulik, "Genetic epidemiology of eating disorders," in *Eating Disorders and Obesity*, ed. Christopher G. Fairburn and Kelly D. Brownell (New York: The Guilford Press, 2002), 238-242.

19. *Ibid*.

20. *Ibid*.

21. Jeffrey DeSarbo, "The Neuroscience of BED Made (somewhat) Easy." Presented at the BEDA annual conference, Nov 6, 2015.

22. Patricia Quinn and Kathleen Nadeau, "Eating disorders and women with ADD," *ADDitude* , 2015, http://www.addiudemag.com/adhd-web/article/2032.html (accessed August 6, 2015); Patricia Quinn and Kathleen Nadeau, *Understanding Women with ADHD* (Silver Springs, MD: Advantage Books, 2002).

23. Michael Strober and Cynthia M. Bulik, "Genetic epidemiology of eating disorders," in *Eating Disorders and Obesity*, ed. Christopher G. Fairburn and Kelly D. Brownell (New York: The Guilford Press, 2002), 238-242.

24. Samuel S. Thatcher, *Polycystic Ovary Syndrome: The hidden epidemic* (Indianapolis, Indiana: Perspectives Press, 2000), p.125-126.

25. Jeffrey DeSarbo, "The Neuroscience of BED Made (somewhat) Easy." Presented at the BEDA annual conference, Nov 6, 2015.

Chapter 5

1. For more information, see Herbert Bensen, *The Relaxation Response* (Berkley, California: The Berkley Publishing Group, 1975). I discuss my use of deep breathing technique in greater detail in chapter 7.

2. Rick Glantz, *Managing Cravings*, (Battle Ground, Washington: Rhea Jacobson Management, 2001), cassette.

Chapter 6

1. University of British Columbia, "Genes predispose some people to focus on the negative," Science Daily (Oct 10, 2013). http://www.sciencedaily.com/releases/2013/10/1310101050539.htm (accessed December 26, 2015).

2. Janet D. Latner and Albert J. Stunkard, "Getting worse: The stigmatization of obese children," *Obesity Research* 11, no. 3 (March 2003), 452-456. This study involved 458 children in the 5th and 6th grades, both boys and girls, and both urban and suburban schools. It included whites (71%), Hispanics (12%), Asian (10%), African Americans (3%), and Native Americans (2%).

3. Stephen Richardson, Norman Goodman, Albert H. Hastorf and Sanford M. Dornbusch, "Cultural uniformity in reaction to physical disabilities," *American Sociological Review* 26, no. 2 (April 1961), 241-247. This study involved 640 children, both boys and girls aged 10-11 and included whites, African Americans, and Puerto Ricans; Janet D. Latner and Albert J. Strunkard, "Getting worse: The stigmatization of obese children," *Obesity Research* 11, no. 3 (March 2003), 452-456.

4.   R. M. Puhl and Kelly D. Brownell, "Psychosocial origins of obesity stigma: Toward changing a powerful and pervasive bias," *Obesity Reviews* 4 (2003), 213-227.

5.   Michaela Gulemetova, Darrel Drury, and Catherine P. Bradshaw. "National Education Association Bullying Study," *Colleagues* 6, Iss. 2, Article 11 (2011).

6.   R. M. Puhl and Kelly D. Brownell, "Psychosocial origins of obesity stigma: Toward changing a powerful and pervasive bias," *Obesity Reviews* 4 (2003), 213-227.

7.   Rebecca Puhl and Kelly D. Brownell, "Stigma, discrimination, and obesity," in *Eating Disorders and Obesity*, ed. Christopher G. Fairburn and Kelly D. Brownell (New York: The Guilford Press, 2002), 108-112.

8.   Foster, Gary D. et al. "Primary care physicians' attitudes about obesity and its treatment." *Obesity Research, 11* (October 2003), 1168-1177.

9.   C.S. Crandall and K.L. Schiffhauer, "Anti-fat prejudice, beliefs, values, and American culture," *Obesity Research* 6 (1998), 458-460; C.S.Crandall, "Prejudice against fat people: Ideology and self-interest," *Journal of Psychology and Social Psychology* 66 (1994), 882-984; R. M. Puhl and Kelly D. Brownell, "Psychosocial origins of obesity stigma: Toward changing a powerful and pervasive bias," *Obesity Reviews* 4 (2003), 213-227.

10.   Rebecca Puhl and Kelly D. Brownell, "Stigma, discrimination, and obesity," in *Eating Disorders and Obesity*, ed. Christopher G. Fairburn and Kelly D. Brownell (New York: The Guilford Press, 2002), 108-112; R. M. Puhl and Kelly D. Brownell, "Psychosocial origins of obesity stigma: Toward

changing a powerful and pervasive bias," *Obesity Reviews* 4 (2003), 213-227.

11. Elizabeth Pratt, Christy F. Telch, Erich W. Lavouvie, G. Terrence Wilson and W. Steward Agras, "Perfectionism in women with binge eating disorder," *International Journal of Eating Disorders 29,* no 2 (March 2001), 177-186.

12. For more information refer to Albert Ellis, *Overcoming Destructive Beliefs, Feelings, and Behavior: New Directions for Rational Emotive Behavior* (Amherst, New York: Prometheus, 2001) and other works by Ellis. For a more theoretical discussion see Aaron Beck, *Cognitive Behavior of Substance Abuse* (New York: Guilford Press, 1999) and other works by Beck.

13. K.A. Brownley, N.A. Berkman, J.A. Sedway, K.N. Lohr and C.M. Bulik, "Binge eating disorder treatment: A systematic review of randomized clinical trials." *International Journal of Eating Disorders*, 40 (2007), 337-348; Denise E. Wilfley, "Psychological treatment of binge eating disorder," in *Eating Disorders and Obesity*, ed. Christopher G. Fairburn and Kelly D. Brownell (New York: The Guilford Press, 2002), 350-353.

14. Cynthia M. Bulik, *Binge Control: A Compact Recovery Guide* (Create Space Independent Publishing Platform, 2015); Victor R. Pendelton, Ken G. Goodrich, Walker S. Poston, Rebecca S. Reeves and John P. Foreyt, "Exercise augments the effects of cognitive behavioral therapy in treatment of binge eating," *International Journal of Eating Disorders* 31, no. 2 (March 2002), 172-173.

Chapter 7

1.   K. M. Flegal, B.K. Kit, H. Orpana and B.I. Graubard, "Association of all-cause mortality with overweight and obesity using standard body mass index categories: A systematic review and meta-analysis." *Journal of the American Medical Association*, 309, no.1 (2013), 71-82.

2.   *Ibid.*

3.   National Weight Loss Registry. http://www.nwcr.ws/Research/default.htm (accessed July 26. 2015). For a full discussion of other findings in the National Weight Loss Registry also see: James Hill and Rena Wing, "A focus on obesity, Part II," *The Permanente Journal* 7 (Summer 2003).

4.   K. Jason Crandall and Patricia A Eisenman, "Physical exercise: A treatment option for binge eating disorder?" *Women in Sport & Physical Activity Journal* 10, no. 2 (Fall 2001), 95-120; Victor R. Pendelton, Ken G. Goodrich, Walker S. Poston, Rebecca S. Reeves and John P. Foreyt, "Exercise augments the effects of cognitive behavioral therapy in treatment of binge eating," *International Journal of Eating Disorders* 31, no. 2 (March 2002): 172-184.

5.   Cynthia M. Bulik and Nadine Taylor, *Runaway Eating* (New York: Rodale, 2005), 59.

6.   Cynthia M. Bulik, "Anxiety, depression, and eating disorders," in *Eating Disorders and Obesity*, ed. Christopher G. Fairburn and Kelly D. Brownell (New York: The Guilford Press, 2002), 193-196.

7.   James A. Blumenthal et al, "Effects of exercise training on older patients with major depression," *Archives of Internal Medicine* 159 (Oct 1999), 2349-2356.

8.   Carlos M. Grilo, "Binge eating disorder," in *Eating Disorders and Obesity*, ed. Christopher G. Fairburn and Kelly D. Brownell (New York: The Guilford Press, 2002), 178-182.

9.   Lynne Hasselmann, "Ten simple ways to achieve a healthy weight," *Healthplus*, November 9, 2005, http://vanderbiltowc.wellsource.com/ (accessed November 9, 2005).

10. R. Leproult, G. Copinschi, O. Buxton, and E. Van Cauter, "Sleep loss results in an elevation of cortisol levels the next morning," *Sleep* 865-70 (Oct 20 1997).

11. *The Journal of Sleep* (2005).

12. E. Van Cauter, *Annals of Internal Medicine* (December 7 2004); Turek, F. and J. Bass, *Archives of Internal Medicine* (Jan, 2005).

13. K.A. Brownley, N.A. Berkman, J.A. Sedway, K.N. Lohr and C.M. Bulik, "Binge eating disorder treatment: A systematic review of randomized clinical trials." *International Journal of Eating Disorders*, 40 (2007), 337-348; Denise E. Wilfley, "Psychological treatment of binge eating disorder," in *Eating Disorders and Obesity*, ed. Christopher G. Fairburn and Kelly D. Brownell (New York: The Guilford Press, 2002), 350-353.

14. Cynthia M. Bulik, *Binge Control: A Compact Recovery Guide* (CreateSpace Independent Publishing Platform, 2015).

15. *Ibid.*

16. "EMDR: Eye movement desensitization and reprocessing." Web MD. http://www.webmd.com/mental-health/emdr-what-is-it (accessed Oct 8, 2015).

17. Jeffrey DeSarbo, "The Neuroscience of BED Made (somewhat) Easy." Presented at the BEDA annual conference, Nov 6, 2015.

18. James Greenblatt, "The Great Medication Controversy: Vyvanse and the Emergence of BED treatment Drugs." Presented at the BEDA annual conference, Nov 6, 2015.

19. For more on this subject, see Herbert Bensen, *The Relaxation Response* (Berkley, California: The Berkley Publishing Group, 1975).

20.   Ruth Quillian-Wolever, interview by Hilda Dulin Lee, November 20, 2003, Durham, North Carolina, Duke Center for Integrative Medicine.

21. M.M Delmonte, "Meditation and anxiety reduction: A literature review," *Clinical Psychology Review* 5 (1985), 91-102; J.D. Teasdale, Z. Segal and J.M. Williams, "How does cognitive therapy prevent depressive relapse and why should attentional control (mindfulness) training help," *Behavioral Research and Training* 33 (1995), 25-39; J. Kabat-Zinn, A. Massion, J. Kristeller, et all, "Effectiveness of a meditation-based stress reduction intervention treatment of anxiety disorders," *American Journal of Psychiatry* 149 (1992), 936-943. Also see Robert Scaer, *The Body Bears the Burden: Trauma, Dissociation, and Disease* (New York: The Haworth Medical Press, 2001).

22. P. Gelderloos, K.G. Walton, D.W. Orme-Johnson and C.N. Alexander, "Effectiveness of the transcendental

meditation program in preventing and treating substance abuse: A review," *International Journal of Addictions* 26 (1991), 293-325.

Chapter 8

1.   Robert Browing, "Andrea del Sarto," Poetry Foundation (2015), http://www.poetryfoundation.org/poem/173001 (accessed July 27, 2015).

2.   Elizabeth Pratt, Christy F. Telch, Erich W. Lavouvie, G. Terrence Wilson and W. Steward Agras, "Perfectionism in women with binge eating disorder," *International Journal of Eating Disorders 29,* no 2 (March 2001), 177-186; Cynthia M. Bulik and Nadine Taylor, *Runaway Eating* (New York: Rodale, 2005), 60.

3.   Albert Bandura, *Self-Efficacy: The Exercise of Control* (New York: W. H. Freeman, 1997), 13.

4.   David Dunkley, Kirk R. Blankstein, Robin M. Masheb and Carlos M. Grilo, "Personal standards and evaluative concerns dimensions of 'clinical' perfectionism," *Behavioral Research and Therapy* 44, no. 1 (Jan 2006).

Chapter 9   No chapter notes

Chapter 10

1.   I could not locate information on this particular study, but there are many excellent books and papers on the use of healing visualization. The works of researchers such as Carl and Stephanie Simonton, Jeanne Achterberg, Bernie Siegel, Larry Dorsey, Norman Cousins, and Peggy Huddleston are a

starting point for information on the use of relaxation and visualization as it relates to medical care.

2.   Carl G. Jung, *The Portable Jung*, Ed. Joseph Campbell (New York: Penguin Books, 1976).

3.   Mark Cartwright, "Minoan Civilization," *Ancient History Encyclopedia*, Sept 2009, http://www.ancient.eu/Minoan_Civilization/ (accessed July 7, 2010); "The Minoan Civilization of Crete," *Bbc.co.uk*, October 3, 2002. http://www.bbc.co.uk/dna/h2g2/A765146/ (accessed September 3, 2006).

4.   Mary Renault, *The Bull from the Sea* (New York: Pantheon Books, 1962).

5.   Mark Cartwright, "Minoan Civilization," *Ancient History Encyclopedia*, Sept 2009, http://www.ancient.eu/Minoan_Civilization/ (accessed July 7, 2010); "The Minoan Civilization of Crete," *Bbc.co.uk*, October 3, 2002. http://www.bbc.co.uk/dna/h2g2/A765146/ (accessed September 3, 2006).

6.   Mary Renault, *The Bull from the Sea* (New York: Pantheon Books, 1964).

Chapter 11

1.   For more information on how mind-body techniques can be used in preparation for surgery, see Peggy Huddleston, *Heal Faster, Prepare for Surgery: A Guide of Mind-Body Techniques* (Cambridge, Massachusetts: Angel River Press, 2012).

Chapter 12

1.   Mary Caroline Richards, *Centering: In Pottery, Poetry, and the Person* (Middletown, Connecticut: Wesleyan University Press, 1962), 9.

Additional Reading List

In addition to the references listed in the Chapter Notes, I recommend the following to those interested in reading further on topics in this book:

Bledsoe, Bill (2004). *Battle of the Binge*. New York: Bledsoe and Bledsoe Publishing House.

Bly, Robert (1988). *A Little Book on the Human Shadow*. San Francisco: Harper Collins.

Brownell, Kelly D. and Katherine Battle Horgen (2004). *Food Fight*. New York: McGraw-Hill Companies.

Bulik, Cynthia M (2009). *Crave: Why You Binge and How to Stop*. New York: Walker.

Bulik, Cynthia M. (2013). *Midlife Eating Disorder: Your Journey to Recover*. New York: Walker.

Bulik, Cynthia M. (2011). *Woman in the Mirror: How to Stop Confusing What You Look Like with Who You Are*. New York:Walker.

Bulik, Cynthia M. and Nadine Taylor (2005). *Runaway Eating*. New York: Rodale.

Fairburn, Christopher G. and Kelly D. Brownell, eds. (2002). *Eating Disorders and Obesity*. New York: The Guilford Press.

Fairburn, Christopher G. (1995). *Overcoming Binge Eating*. New York: The Guilford Press.

Ford, Debbie (1998). *The Dark Side of the Light Chasers*. New York: Riverhead Books.

Jamison, Kay Redfield (1995). *An Unquiet Mind*. New York: A.A. Knopf.

Pfeiffer, Richard H. (2002). *The Real Solution: Binge/Compulsive Eating Workbook*. New York: Growth Publishing.

Roth, Geneen (1984). *Breaking Free from Compulsive Eating*. New York: Signet Book.

Roth, Geneen (1982). *Feeding the Hungry Heart*. New York: Signet Group.

Roth, Geneen (1991). *When Food is Love*. New York: Plume Book.

Scaer, Robert C. (2001). *The Body Bears the Burden: Trauma, Dissociation, and Disease*. New York: The Haworth Medical Press.

THE AUTHOR

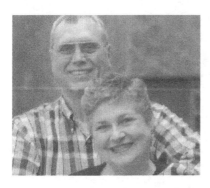 **Hilda Dulin Lee**, a dentist and writer, calls both North Alabama and Western North Carolina home. She attended the University of Alabama in Huntsville where she received her BA degree in literature and did post-graduate work in the sciences. She then attended dental school and received her Doctor of Dental Medicine (DMD) degree. She owned and managed a successful dental practice, taught at her dental school, and conducted seminars and private consultations on practice management. After practicing dentistry for many years, she made a decision that would alter the direction of her life: she sold her beloved dental practice and enrolled in graduate school at the University of North Carolina in Asheville. There she received a Master of Liberal Arts degree in which she combined the study of creative writing and binge eating disorder. *In the Labyrinth of Binge Eating* is her first full-length book. At present, she is working on a collection of personal essays as well as a book about her family's search for the still-missing body of her half-brother, Dan, who was killed in the Korean War. Hilda was selected as a national finalist in Sequestrum's 2015 New Writers Award. Her cottage in Western North Carolina is her favorite place to write. She shares life with her husband, Glenn, who has been the abiding love of her life for more than fifty years. They have two children and eight grandchildren. Her hobbies include genealogy, bridge, and of course reading and writing.

Made in the USA
Charleston, SC
27 June 2016